Plan

CW01086701

Is Mental Health Really 1 ___ _... End All Of
Our Dreams? Or Are We Just Deluded?

Jamie Kershaw

chipmunkapublishing
the mental health publisher

Jamie Kershaw

Published by
Chipmunkapublishing
PO Box 6872
Brentwood
Essex CM13 1ZT
United Kingdom

http://www.chipmunkapublishing.com

Chipmunkapublishing gratefully acknowledge the support of Arts Council England.

Plan 103f

Acknowledgements

Thanks to Paul and Jason at Chipmunkapublishing for making the project a reality, Mum and Dad for always being there for me, Chris and Emma for spurring me along over the years, Oliver and Cameron, Jonny, Jonty, Chris B, Sam, Alan, Tony, Martin – keep it up guys! Margaret Allen, Simon Muir, David 'Live' Ives, Alex Boorman, Scarlett Britten, David and Rose Goodwin, David and Jill Bowman, John and Helen Dean, Stacy Stone, Scarborough Rethink, Mark Bushnell, Hugh Dias and Tim Anderson for teaching me English in earlier years, Dr Myogorosy, Matthew Havenhand, Michelle Turner aka Micha bear, Alida Brown, Kath Sands, Paul Wilson, Colin, Sally, Kathleen, and everyone else – you know who you are - for being there when it mattered most. Thankyou all!

Jamie is 30 years old, born 1978, male, and currently lives in Scarborough, North Yorkshire, UK with fiancée. In 2007 he graduated from Hull University, East Yorkshire, and qualified as a B.A. from the Business School. Whilst there he trained for and completed the Paris Marathon in April 2006 in 3 hrs 25 mins and still has the worn out shoes to prove it! He has also bungee jumped, white-water rafted, and firewalked. He sat and passed 10 GCSEs and 4 A-levels at Durham School 1995/97.

However, in September 1998 he was diagnosed with schizophrenia aged 20, and over a ten year period has had three significant hospital admissions. With medications ranging from Depixol, Haloperidol, Lorazepam Olazapine, Rispiradone, Quetiapine, Abilify, and Clopixol this condition has been monitored and stabilised over the years. The script for Plan 103f was written whilst living as a bachelor in Scarborough Rethink supported accommodation. Some of the inspirations were taken from actual experience, some from broken dreams, and others from the imagination. There were over 50 interviews conducted with independent branch cafés to compile details for The Flaming Squirrels!

Jamie is something of a semi-professional pianist and occasionally plays in public for an audience. His interests in music have been ongoing all his life, also playing limited guitar, viola and harmonica.

Whilst on the degree course he spent one year in Canada on an exchange based at Dalhousie University, Halifax, Nova Scotia – and also travelled independently across to Vancouver and back again by Greyhound bus, train, ferry and plane.

He has also travelled in European countries including Austria, France, Germany, Spain, Czech Republic, the Netherlands, and Norway by train, coach, car, and plane and has a certain grasp of French, Spanish and Russian language. Plan 103f is his first novel.

Plan 103f

Synopsis

Set in a two year timeframe 2010-2012, aiming towards the London 2012 Olympic Games, seven principal characters in their twenties with very different interests and lifestyles come together, experiencing trials, tribulations, successes and failures, heartaches, romance, and learn to pull themselves together despite their discontent.

Tim Richardson (21) is a Triathlete hoping to compete and win a title at the London 2012 Olympic Games. Can he become Olympic champion? He also excels at BMX biking and is coached by Ben Williams (29), an Ethics Professor with a PhD - based in Scarborough. Ben is the most mature of the seven characters. He becomes the owner of a cocker spaniel called Pépé who is admired by Suzanna Jeffries (22). Suzanna is a marathon athlete and triathlete. These two start to see each other after a long and troublesome intervention by her brother Shane Jeffries (24) who is neurotically obsessed with his younger sister to the point of physicality against potential suitors. Shane is a 3rd degree taekwondo blackbelt coach, and marathon runner who participates in the London marathon. His other self holds an interest in Physics and secretly hankers for the Nobel Prize in later life.

Alex Davies (32) is in effect 'the boss'. Alex owns a restaurant called "Collage", and goes on to open a café called "The Flaming Squirrels". Suzanna Jeffries is a waitress in both places as the story progresses. These two venues are often used as locations for the seven 'crew' members to hang out and catch up with each other. Alex is married to Melanie, and they have a five year old daughter called Fiona. The other characters always show great respect towards Alex Davies.

Charlie Morris (25) is an entrepreneur who goes on to establish a local tropical fish shop having written his entire business blueprint whilst serving time in a mental hospital with an ASBO for assaulting his father who denied him the necessary encouragement to start out in business. Whilst on the ward he meets Claire Halls (23) who attempted suicide by overdose and is a struggling singer-songwriter. Was this attempt anything to do with her friend

Megan's husbands death? She springs back to life because of Charlie and forms a folk-rock band called 'Seachimp'. Claire is lead singer and acoustic guitarist. The band win a recording contract after they win a local battle of the bands competition and go on a UK tour. Claire and Charlie get married and have a baby called Luke.

There are 18 chapters in total tracing their experiences over the two year period. Good and bad, happy and sad, for richer or for poorer, *Plan 103f* demonstrates how you can reach for your dreams and still need to make new dreams along the way. The novel is set in various locations including Scarborough, London and Scotland.

The fiction/non-fiction element is intended to make it more believable. There is sex, blood, romance, love, money, enterprise, Olympism, and the story winds up with the seven 'crew' members in Alex's establishment 'Collage', evaluating everything they have been through together in this period of time.

The seven principal characters could be said to represent different aspects of the author's own character, broken dreams, and failed experiences. Perhaps representing multiple personalities within the author, thus enabling the realisation of experiences that were otherwise unattainable.

Chapter 1
Exposition

There was something of the constant renaissance about him. As he had lined up to the water's edge that day in London, Tim Richardson had his sights on the Gold. All thoughts of failure eluded him. Standing there at the start line he was trained to win, to win an Olympic title. Could he now defy the odds and become a legend in his own right?

Now in the year 2012 he was able to do everything he had ever trained for and dreamed about. With no further time for reflection it was all down to race day and his experience to determine what could be done. That would remain to be seen, within two short hours. For now, he was on his own and in the zone. Could the hard slog of the previous four years be vindicated?

Life was not always that easy for the others, either; for Alex, he had founded a restaurant and coffee house in this period, and had appreciated the value of working and studying hard without expectation of luck alone. He recognised that good luck would come with the correct application of preparation and perseverance if he could stick it out.

Both Charlie and Alex had found their niche, their passion, prior to which, there had been at least a notion of what was to come; maybe an inkling of an idea on a piece of paper, or a germ of an idea just waiting for an opportunity to flourish. Both had been willing to nurture the original concept and do the right thing time after time in order to progress towards their current day result. This had been no mistake. They had worked hard and deserved the outcome.

Charlie Morris was now married with a three year old son. He had developed an idea for a tropical fish shop in the local town. He had really struggled, but owing to the words of Roy Ash, he had persisted: "An entrepreneur tends to bite off a little more than he can chew, hoping he'll quickly learn how to chew it".

As well as this, he had learnt that "the best reason to start an organization is to make meaning; to create a product or service to make the world a better place." Charlie had intended to do so, just as Guy Kawasaki had said.

Alex and Charlie were one of a kind; both giving life to an original concept, which had come into being through nothing less than hard graft and a useful support network, working in their favour. A mechanism, if you like, that got them into play. Charlie had experienced life from the touch line some years earlier, but had determined to make an idea a reality.

With the good fortune of stumbling across Claire Halls and saving her life, Charlie had found a great purpose and reason to contribute. As Debbi Fields had said: "The important thing is not being afraid to take a chance. Remember, the greatest failure is to not try." Charlie had certainly tried at the best of times since he met Claire.

Thomas Edison had famously declared that "Genius is 1% inspiration, and 99% perspiration." They all knew that. This was just the beginning, and they needed to consolidate a few facts; facts that would take them on a journey of discovery and realisation amongst many unfolding events along the way.

Alex was not alone in his venture, he had a wife Melanie and a young daughter Fiona to look after. He had been something of a role model to Charlie throughout his darkest hour. Alex had shed light on a difficult time for him. Were it not for Alex, Charlie may have even dropped his intention, without ever seeking fulfilment.

As well as Tim, Alex, Claire and Charlie, there were the siblings, Shane and Suzanna Jeffries. Both were young twenty-somethings doing their own thing, going to work and keeping fit. They got on despite being related by family name and were a key part of the crew through and through. They had helped Tim get so far with his athletic career. Both had been training alongside him at some point in time.

There was also a more mature figure in his thirties, Benjamin Williams. He had been selected for a professorial post at the local campus round about the year 2008 and had immersed himself in the goings on of the job. It was his first post since qualifying some time beforehand. A bit lonely, maybe, but fully occupied with his work. He had come from the South so the rest of the crew took a while to accept him amongst themselves. There was no turning back the clock anyway, not for Ben, or any of them. They had come to know one another as a consequence of a series of events, not least of which was the prospect of an Olympic Champion.

Tim had been building up to the Games for many years, consciously since he was about fourteen. It had been a dream for him. Never easy, never handed on any kind of platter, never something to take lightly for him, he had been working hard throughout this time.

He was seventeen when the Beijing Olympics took place, still too young, many people thought. Only, for some such as Tom Daley, there was talent present from a very young age, so nothing could be ruled out entirely, of course. The event was still fresh in his mind as he participated and got the results in numerous local meets. Tim was a triathlete. He had watched as Alistair Brownlee made an incredible run at Beijing, but was beaten to the medal table. The fact of an Olympian at all was inspiring enough for him.

Tim sat thinking about what Walt Disney had promised the world in the 20th Century: "If you can dream it, you can do it". Alex Davies had words of his own to add to this. He had known Tim for over five years by now, and had known that his high expectations had been the key to everything he had ever accomplished since then, for better or for worse.

All the while, the Jeffries' siblings were eager to assist in any form of training regime. Shane practised triathlon and taekwondo; he also had Olympic dreams going on, and would often be present at the local pool or on his bike to train alongside Tim. Suzanna too; she would swim in the same pool on a morning, before the masses arrived.

Whereas Tim, Shane and Suzanna were all fighting fit, their local guru – Alex Davies – was purely an entrepreneur. He had no personal interest invested in the athletics track. Although always keen to learn of their results via Suzanna, whom he had employed at his hospitality venues, he would take it all on board and mull it over in his mind along with many other items.

Alex had been married to Melanie for a good five years by now and they had a young infant daughter whom they had called Fiona. She was on the verge of starting school soon. They had hoped to keep their ventures in the family and make careful selection as to whom they would employ. Therefore Suzanna Jeffries had been lucky indeed to be selected to work there.

There were no worries with her, as both parties knew exactly where they stood and they had alternative agendas to keep as well, such as an amateur athletics career and coaching for her, and family to feed for him. Melanie didn't mind that Suzanna was employed to work at Collage, the restaurant.

As Richard Bach said in Illusions: "Rarely do members of one family grow up under the same roof. The bond that links your true family is not one of blood, but of respect and joy in each other's life". For Alex, he would shortly learn the truth of this as he continued to run his enterprise in his own way. There was only one Alex Davies, after all.

As for Claire and Charlie, their lives had undergone a remarkable transition between 2010 and 2012. A real down and out beginning, full of desperation, misery, despair, and isolation had become a fulfilling relationship with high times for all. They had not been alone in this transformational quest, however. The likes of Alex, Ben and the three athletes had been an integral part of it for them. They were all a unit of a kind, the crew.

Now in 2012 Claire was happy, a bestselling recording artist, still lead singer in the folk-rock band Seachimp, Luke's mum, Charlie's wife and something of a traveller/bon viveuse. There had been the opportunity to tour during this time.

Charlie Morris was still the entrepreneur, like Alex. He had conceived his business idea in 2010 whilst locked away for a while, and written up the entire blueprint in this time. Having regained his freedom and made the right approaches, his business had come into being and he now ran a successful tropical fish shop called Fish4U!

His clients would come from all angles at the best of times, especially including fish for restaurants, hotel lobbies, hairdressers' shops and people's living rooms.

Having been through all that, what now lay ahead for them? For Tim, he was anticipating Gold at the London Olympics 2012. There was to be no disappointment as he had made it onto the winners' podium many times before in various meets. The BOA declared him a true ambassador for the sport, and were keen to follow his achievements for the next three Games to come. He was young enough to continue on this line of endeavour for quite some time yet.

Looking ahead, nobody fully knew what to expect, least of all did anyone expect to have to go back through their personal hell that they had since moved away from. Ben had related their traumas to Dante's 'Divine Comedy', or Milton's 'Paradise Lost'. "Through me is the way to the sorrowful city. Through me is the way to eternal suffering. Through me is the way to join the lost people. Abandon all hope, all ye who enter here!" (Dante Alighieri). Or, "There is no greater pain than to remember a happy time when one is in misery."

Claire had been in that position of realising her strengths to be less so, even though present. Undervalued, uncherished and unloved until Charlie came along and turned the whole thing round in a very short period of time. He was her knight in shining armour, the conquering hero who won her heart. He had reignited her soul with reason to live, and motive to contribute.

There was a world out there waiting her recognitions, attentions, and divine inspirations. Many people appreciated the band's music and would nominate themselves as number one fans on the website. Seachimp had pulled through so much over the years and were going from strength to strength. Nothing could stop them now, and Claire Halls was the commander of the ship, the captain of the deck. Charlie Morris stood by her as the band grew.

Milton had written: "For who would lose, though full of pain, this intellectual being, those thoughts that wander through eternity, to perish rather, swallowed up and lost in the wide womb of uncreated night, devoid of sense and motion?"

He also wrote: "The strongest and fiercest spirit that fought in heaven; now fiercer by despair: his trust was with the eternal to be deemed equal in strength, and rather than be less, cared not to be at all" (Paradise Lost).

Charlie too had a direction, a venture to deal with. This was his bread and butter. Selling tropical fish to local buyers. Not to eat, mind, more to witness living in a tank, speculating on whether or not any of their existence actually entered their own memory capacity. For some, a tropical fish was a moment's entertainment, but for Charlie it was his lifeblood.

At this moment in time his entire prerogative was to sell the blighters, and frequently at that. So long as there was custom for his shop, that is what counted most for him. He had been forwarded as regional entrepreneur at one point for his new venture's success. There was plenty of advertising: word-of-mouth, yellow pages, library, hotel lobbies, satisfied customers, Yorkshire Coast Radio, novelty assets to the area, etc. He was happy and grateful to be acknowledged in these ways by others. So long as Fish4U! was getting a fair share of the limelight, that is what counted for him.

Claire would visit him during the daytime, and occasionally help out in the shop. He was on the verge of some sort of partnership with another pet shop in the area. Prior to this he had been a sole trader. A small business, but with an attractive and unique selling point: Why go to the Caribbean, when the Caribbean can come to you?

There was, at least, an air of satisfaction about the tag line. People liked their far away places, and the travel agents could vouch for that every year. So at least they had some form of creature comfort in stock for those who wanted.

Charlie had less contact with Shane and Suzanna, although they were all in on the crew thing. Meeting at Collage, Alex's place, especially, was their main point of contact. Shane could be a moody bugger on occasion, sometimes without forecast, or conscious intent. He had a naturally predatory air about him - something of the lion stalking the zebra. All perfectly in tune with the savannah, but it could be distressing for some.

For example, Suzanna, his sister, would often be his sole means of communication for days on end. This made them bond, but they never really progressed anything on the evolutionary scale, unlike Charlie or Alex, who had evolved dramatically by now. As Darwin indicated, the survival of the fittest was in process; or maybe the survival of the wily, like a coyote on the prairie, or a hyena in the wilderness.

Tim, Shane, Suzanna, Ben, Alex, Charlie, and Claire were a special unit together. Part of their own culture in a way. They would meet up for recaps, updates and new outcomes. Always willing to dispense advice where necessary, these seven characters had become closely knit over the last five years, starting from scratch.

Just as a lounge was home to any of them, a result would be shared as though an integral part of all of their doing. Nobody could take too much credit on their own for an outcome. There had to be a bit of give and take, a little bit of this and that, something of a united state of consequence, something like Che Guevara attempting to unite the countries of Latin America into a United State. Only, the crew were on a more intimate level. They actually knew one another and the revolution was of a different kind. More of a humanistic basis. Che Guevara rebelled on a massive scale, so much so that he was upheld as the revolutionary of the time. Charlie and Alex were New Venture Creators, money generators, generation makers, holistic divinators, and they knew what to do within their own sphere of endeavour.

This brought a sense of peace to them at this point in time, as they were together reflecting on the period just gone.

"I was thinking", said Alex, "it's a good job somebody could".
"Yeah", replied Charlie, "it's definitely a good job".

They remained reflective for a moment. Then Ben piped up: "Well, there's nothing like the real thing".
"That's history now, mate. We're all blown away by the facts", Ben continued.

Suzanna chipped in at this point: "and I bet there's more to come yet, is there not, Mister?" referring to Alex's high standards.

They were less for creeds, more for deeds, talking about action and results rather than hyperbole alone. Their most recent actions had brought them all together once again. Collage was fairly quiet at this point, so it seemed like a good time to meet there and actually pay each other full attention all the while. There was nothing worse than being ignored, well ok, maybe one thing - and that would be not even being talked about at all; either up front or behind closed doors.

These people had made explicit commitment to pay attention to one another's details since they became a community of a kind. Sometimes there just was not enough time to go around for them, other times there was just not enough happening for them. Either way, they never got on each other's wick for too long.

There was always the 'Sheriff' to deal with, i.e., who was boss. At the best of times, Alex was the unappointed chief – probably because it was his place they always met at; the happening venue. There was no real discrepancy about this unspoken elect. The crew seemed to appreciate all the goings on, anyway.

"Howzat for efficiency?" asked Claire, as the drinks were brought on a tray for them all.

There was lemonade, white wine spritzer, Tetley's, freshly squeezed orange juice, white coffee, Kronenbourg, and Appletise for them all to go at. They clinked their glasses and proceeded to drink in regular sips, all the while wondering what to say.

"Prometheus stole fire from the Gods", uttered Ben philosophically. "He was doing the people a great service, an enormous favour by doing so. Everyone knew that," he went on.

"But the Gods chained him to a mountain for the eagles to peck out his liver by day", interjected Suzanna. "His liver grew back by night for the eagles to eat the next day", she said knowledgeably.

Ben commended her for continuing his story.

"So, what's the point of that illustration, then, Ben?" asked Charlie.

"Well, I mean to say, you can do the people a service, but if you're messing with the divine, you'd better stand guard."

They nodded sagely at his wisdom. Then Suzanna inquired "But what if the Gods liked the people as well?"

"They are another breed. Although some would say that modern man in a suit and tie is the manifestation of God – smart, fit, strong, quick, intelligent, affluent, together, and true."

"My, that's interesting", Suzanna commented conclusively.

There was a bit of sage chin-rubbing going on at the table by now, and Ben was satisfied to have provoked some thought. He was renowned for adding a little intellect to the modus operandi of the time, without being funny about it.

Alex always appreciated a wise yarn in his establishments. It all added up to a more wholesome experience. On one wall there was a series of quotes by famous authors, philosophers, scientists, poets, and other great minds of the previous few centuries. "It ain't Shakespeare", he quipped, "but you know what it means, at least."

Ben laughed at that: "Too much writing was not Shakespeare, so one simply had to contend with a lesser creation. How do you think Beethoven got so big in the 19th Century?" He had been one of fourteen siblings; at least Ben had a chance of being noticed without worrying about his own siblings' contention. He had none.

Alex, too, was an only child, as was Charlie. They all had common ground here. Shane and Suzanna could appreciate their position by the simple fact of being from the same family, the Jeffries. This was not their doing. They were born, so they lived. More an act of destiny; fate in the making. Nothing would ever change that for them.

Charlie was relieved to have stumbled upon Claire some years earlier. Were it not for him, their entire relationship may never have occurred. No record contract, no CD's, no tour, no name. Just abject ignominy.

As it was, they did meet and that sparked up a rekindling of faith within the human spirit. A spark had caused a flame, and the flame had been burning brightly for years now. Others were happy to see to it that this fire was well stoked, like a November bonfire.

As for their son, little Luke, well he still had no real concept of all that had passed. Didn't need to, and certainly there were no expectations that he should. Still too young. He was a bundle of cuddles and laughter for them. Just walking on his own two feet by now and speaking some select first words. He brought joy to Claire just by being there. By the very act of existing.

Their addition to the crew had come about in a round-about kind of way. But more on that later. For now, Luke Morris was the youngest member of them all. But by no means least.

Ben had been looking after his dog for a good few years and was well into the swing of things. It had taken a whole lot of persuasion and moral debate whether to acquire a canine companion or not, but in the end he had elected to go for it and get a lifelong friend – something that had been lacking in his life up until then. That point caused action, and the consequence was a canine companion for life. Tim got on with him more as mentor, but the dog caused a point of interest. Alex found a few difficulties with Ben's dog trying to get into Collage. This was a moot point to be continuously reviewed as they approached the door.

Tim was not just local news. As well as being Alex's hero, he was a regular feature in line with the British Olympic Association. Various interviews and podcasts had been made with Tim starring. It was all available for review online and in the magazine publications. Tim Richardson was big news.

Were it not for Tim's hero, Tim Don, winning the world championships, many people would probably not have heard of Triathlon in the UK. Since that event, the sport had become more a household word, with stars known to many. By the time the London Games came, Tim Richardson had become a household name, with expectations for great things to come.

The event had turned his life upside down – only in a great way, coming from all obscurity with a fit body, to a regular member recognised by all. This rapid transition had made him more aware of all that he had never known beforehand, all that he had seen, but not yet experienced for himself. His life was on the make, and making him was the body of folk who believed in him. That number was increasingly building up, so much so, that hearing strangers greet him had become a regular occurrence; people wanting a piece of his soul, a piece of his fit body. They wanted his ass on their doorstep.

Would it be rugged, or would it be more levelled? That was something that Tim wondered about. He had come in to land on a level playing field, and there were folk to greet him as he landed. That is all he knew and cared about.

Alex was one of those who had the faith going on. Ben was there from the early days. Wearing a stopwatch at the local meets, he would time Tim (in addition to the official timers). That way, all notes could be compared and contrasted when the runners came home. Ben had logged a series of diaries of all Tim's training details over a five year period. They enjoyed poring over this together to take note of what worked best of all in the long run. How could he improve? How could he become higher, stronger, faster? Citius, Altius , Fortius.

Suzanna, too, had a personal hero. Also a triathlete, Suzanna revered Chrissie Wellington – the 2007 Iron Man Hawaii champion, and World Champion of the time. She was at the top of the tree in this sport, with others having to follow her home. She had met a keen, fit triathlete called Patrick who had been an inspiration, so mentioned the details to Tim when they met.

Tim could whip round the Olympic distance course in under two hours on a good day with little or no wind present. Patrick had a personal best time of two hours eleven minutes which was still in an elite bracket, and would prove faster than the majority.

Chrissie had previously been a Government official in foreign lands prior to winning her title. This furthered Suzanna's interest in her achievements. One day, when she was talking with Tim, they decided to sing the Olympic Anthem for good measure:

> Immortal spirit of antiquity
> Father of the true, beautiful and good
> Descend, appear, shed over us thy light
> Upon this ground and under this sky
> Which has first witnessed thy unperishable fame
>
> Give life and animation to these noble Games!
> Throw wreaths of fadeless flowers to the victors
> In the race and in the strife
> Create in our breasts, hearts of steel!
>
> In thy light, plains, mountains and seas
> Shine in a roseate hue and form a vast temple
> To which all nations throng to adore thee
> Oh immortal spirit of antiquity!

They felt profoundly moved by the lyrics, as they were close to their hearts. Tim had been living the lifestyle of an Olympian for over five years by this point. The direction was steady and definite. He was a brave athlete in many respects.

The five Olympic values universal to all were: sportsmanship, education, exceeding ones expectations, solidarity, peace and happiness   The Olympic Games represented an ideal whose spirit was kept alive by these five values created by the International Olympic Committee (IOC). Sport, culture and respect presented the three pillars of the Olympic ideal. Looking at the values in turn: *Sportsmanship* encouraged each athlete to give better than their best, to strive beyond all known achievement, to not only win the race but, at the same time be graceful in the face of defeat and accept that participation in this race meant experience necessary to gain the edge in the next. Sportsmanship meant knowing how to win even when somebody else was winning.

Education was constant and never ending; always improving, always learning, always evolving, often without realising. Continuously becoming and in doing so, educating others, too.

Exceeding ones expectations in life gave Tim a huge survival guidance, since we were either living or dying, creating or destroying. If we did not build then we died, no matter what the context. We were designed to innovate and by continuously building a new level every day we were thus exceeding our expectations.

Solidarity translated as unity in diversity. The whole world came together for 17 days at a time to celebrate pure achievement. Everybody united over the Olympics.

P*eace and happiness* came from fulfilling lifetime objectives, having come through all manner of challenge on the journey.

Called to achieve certain objectives, and in this case, those who achieved Olympic Gold would surely experience profound peace and happiness. "Higher, faster, stronger!" Athletes *intended* to win the gold, supporters intended to *see* the athletes win the gold, and the organisers intended to *enable* the athletes to win the gold.

The Beijing Games 2008 cost over £22.9bn, the largest and most spectacular Games of all time, and over 10,500 athletes from more than 202 nations were present. It was calculated that 20,200 media representatives worked as journalists to record the event in every detail, which for China meant that in just 17 days, more journalists visited the country than in the entire past 100 years.

The phenomenal growth over the last 30 years saw a cottage industry grow from the 1980 Moscow Games in a financial abyss, to a multi-billion dollar global success, making and breaking media empires, launching and reinvigorating global brands, whilst bringing investment across otherwise distant borders between nations.

Ben had done some research and told Tim that "Olympism is a philosophy of life, exaltation, and combining in a balanced whole the qualities of body, will and mind. Blending sport with culture and education, Olympism seeks to create a way of life based on the joy found in effort, the education, value of and example and respect for universal fundamental ethical principles".

Now presided by Jacques Rogge (the 8th IOC President), elected 16th July 2001. He took over the reins from Juan Antonio Samaranch (Spanish Honorary President for life) who was inducted in the IOC as far back as 1966. Samaranch was chiefly responsible for the 1980-2001 IOC economic turnaround seeing £120,000 become £22.9bn within 30 years.

Tim appreciated Ben's wisdom on the subject and continued to train and adjust his technique where appropriate. He was glad to have such a person as mentor, someone who believed in him for what he could achieve on the course. Suzanna, too, shared his values. They were lucky like that. It was more than pure genetics alone. There was an intellectual-emotional connection as well.

Lord Coe had met Tim prior to the 2012 London Games and his words were full of significance, encouragement, pride, enthusiasm, passion, and determination, intending to drive him onto the winning podium on the day itself.

Tim had seen all of the official DVDs from the Moscow 1980 and Los Angeles 1984 Games to Sydney 2000 and Athens 2004. He had taken dramatic inspiration from the man who did it, who actually won the title in reality. Gold for a Lionheart is the way that Tim saw it.

Maybe he could improve on his own performance and join Lord Coe in that most elite band of athletes. He would have to step up, having already stepped up to a maximum capacity. Perhaps there was no such thing as maximum capacity, as the soul was always developing, the body always metabolising, the mind always ticking, the heart always beating.

In Tim's case, he was prepared to discover a new limit. Where would that be, he wondered. Maybe there would be no limit, an unlimited potential for greater things. He would have to step inside the right shoes for a great adventure. Life's supreme challenges remained for him. He still had the time and still had youth on his side. For all it was worth, there were seven people in the original crew. They all shared a similar commitment.

The ancient prophets could not have put it any clearer. The principles were known right through the centuries past, up to the present day. Just as Ribena berries were giving a critically important lesson about vitamins, Tim, Ben and Suzanna were looking at some serious stuff with a lighter slant to it. They were defying the laws of gravity. By looking to the stars their time on earth was appeased.

Tim was a star in his own right, and there were plenty of people looking out for his name. More than just an athlete, he was a best friend, a role model to the nation, and an educator in doing what he did best – the triathlon. At an earlier age he had been a keen exponent of BMX bike-riding, but that is a story for later. Many occurrences had cropped up owing to this experience.

He stumbled across a Team GB colleague, Vinny, as a direct consequence of this sporting endeavour. Vinny was from up North, near Newcastle, and only really came across Tim during the major meets in the UK. They were buddies on a perennial basis, on the premise that they could meet and compete, train without complaint, and otherwise get on with their own thing in an unbiased manner, without interferences or other niggles to distract them from the main event.

After all, it was the main event that drew everybody like a magnet emitting powerful forces of attraction. People came from all angles just to say they were a part of it. If each soul could be thought of as an iron filing, then the Games was the pulling force, with all the pulling power. London 2012 was the magnet, causing great things to occur in its name. Shenaz Reade had proven a huge inspiration on her BMX at the Beijing Games 2008. Tim had watched.

As they sat reflecting on all the impossibility of such an achievement the thought was still there that he could go that extra mile and capture the title. Suzanna hastened to add that Chrissie Wellington had not been given her title on a silver platter. It had been no bed of roses all the way. There were trials and experimentations to be had, styles to be discovered, techniques to be deployed, and the winning inch to be gained.

Tim could have revelled in his immediate capacity, but he was made of sterner stuff than that. Not one to rest on his laurels, or sit back on his haunches, he had to find a way, every day, to keep in the game, whether by mind or by body or by spirit. Tim Richardson was no slouch.

Alex told him that, as well. If there was a God, then Tim would find out over the years. Claire and Charlie had made good ground since their earlier traumas. It seemed a different world now that they had come into the warmth and light of their people. Both had become able to perform in various guises, and with Alex close at hand to keep them on track, things seemed to be going really well. As for Shane, well, he would keep up the taekwondo and triathlon, whilst studying hard in the Physics lab. He had a lot of respect for those who could get their heads around Quantum Physics. The laws that they uncovered were incredible, the principles of the universe that worked the same for everybody seemed improbable at first, but the more he got into that mode of thinking, the more it made sense.

The crew were in this together, and they were blessed to know this. What had they come through over the years to make it so? What would they go through in the future? Who would they come across, and would anyone else come in on the act?

All these questions, questions of progress and evolution, were in their minds. Ben, Tim, Alex, Shane, Suzanna, Claire, and Charlie were the crew. They had plans – A to Z – that was a given, so surely life would present the greener grass, on the sunny side of the park. What you reap was what you keep. The seeds you sow became the plants you know. This was just the beginning.

Chapter 2
Two years earlier

The year was 2010; it was the springtime, April. The Vancouver Winter Olympic Games had just been. There had been 5,500 athletes representing 80 countries, of which 1,350 paralympic athletes represented 40 countries. 1.6 million spectator tickets had been sold, whilst 10,000 media representatives recorded and documented the events. The Games' security budget extended to $900 million, and the total cost for Vancouver 2010 came to $1.76 billion. The average temperature around the mountains, stadiums, and local area was recorded at 4.8C.

The lucky mascots for Vancouver were Miga, Quatchi, Sumi, and Mukmuk. From the choice of events, Team GB had a number of Gold medal potentials including Zoe Gillings and Ben Kilner (Snowboarding), Sinead and John Kerr (figure-skating), Nicola Minichiello and Gillian Cooke (Bobsleigh), Shelley Rudman (flagbearer and skeleton run), Chemmy Alcott (skiing), Jenna McCorkell (figure skating), Kristian Bromley (men's skeleton), A J Rosen (luge), and the men's curling team captained by David Murdoch. Could Eve Muirhead and the women's Curlers repeat the Gold of 2002 in Salt Lake City captained by Rhona Martin? Amy Williams had become Olympic skeleton champion, and won Team GB's only actual Gold in 30 winter years! Shelley Rudman had provided inspiration for Team GB with her 2006 Turin Silver in the skeleton run. Ed Drake made a very impressionable 33rd place skiing for Team GB. All were still consumed with the 1984 Sarajevo Gold won by Jayne Torvill and Christopher Dean ice-dancing. Their 1994, Lillehammer, Bronze follow-up was equally inspiring.

Other Winter Games events in Vancouver included speed-skating, snowboarding, freestyle skiing, alpine & cross-country skiing, biathlon, ski jumping, bobsleigh, skeleton, luge, ice hockey, and Nordic combined. The Georgian team demonstrated true Olympic spirit despite the death of Nodar Kumaritashvili on a practice luge run prior to the Opening Ceremony. Team Canada ended up dominating the medals table, with 14 Golds, 7 Silvers, and 5 Bronze medals, compared to a German lead in Turin (therefore making up for the earlier Montreal and Calgary Games on Canadian home turf). Notably, the Ice Hockey showed Canadian victory yet again for the men and the women.

Tim Richardson was competing for a place on Team GB as an excellent triathlete, looking ahead to London 2012. However, Charlie Morris was sat in a secure ward for six months. Benjamin Williams had just been offered a first post as Professor. Shane and Suzanna Jeffries were busy keeping fit, and working hard not to fall out all the time. Alex Davies was running his restaurant, and Claire Halls had taken an overdose. Unbeknown to each other at that time, within the space of the forthcoming months their paths were destined to cross.

The thing with Tim was his athletic prowess. Weighing in at 87kg, at 5' 10'', Tim still had his dream going on. He was going for broke. His training was his business. In earlier years, as a teenager he had represented the county and won his races on a bike. He had completed some fast triathlons and seemed multi-talented to many. Good on a BMX as well, he could pull stunts, grip the imagination of his peers, and ride a fair session on the course. But he suffered at the mercy of his cynics' hands.

Only one member in his entire family history had ever had a record of athletic success: his grandpa Billy, who ran an Olympic marathon in the 1960 Rome Summer Games. He hadn't made the top 10 even but he was there. Tim's parents would say "why don't you go to college like all the other smart kids? Train to be a doctor or a lawyer?" Tim would absent himself onto his bike within a heart beat and off he would ride, training again. This elusive pattern concerned them. And his arguments puzzled them.

Tim had learnt some valuable life lessons from this period in his life, and grown both older and wiser for it, even though still a stripling. With time to prepare ahead of him he set to reading about his athletic heroes, and his cycling champions. The Tour de France, the World Championships, La Vuelta d'Espana, Il Giro d'Italia, Olympic Games Past, Present and yet to be. He had fired up about the London Summer Games 2012, all the more because of the Team GB success at Beijing 2008, hauling 19 Gold medals in the various sports. He still struggled to get others to believe in him fully. He found it difficult to find somebody else to share his youthful enthusiasms. He was on his own here for a while. Until Ben Williams came into the equation he would be in a state of constant frustration.

He once yelled at his parents as they queried his dedication: "I *NEED* my bike! Where's my training schedule? I *NEED* to get out there. I have a dream. My bike is my life!" He meant business.

On the other hand, Ben William's years of academia had instilled some critical values into him. He could see perfectly clearly what Tim was on with from the safety of the sidelines. Ben had no qualms in sharing his values with Tim. Right from day one he and Tim had an understanding. Although to some people, Ben was misunderstood by them. Easily done, given his tendency to soliloquize overtly, irrespective of time or location. Tim could make good sense of him anyhow.

As well as his teaching, Ben was something of an author. He wrote about heavy-duty stuff; ethics, philosophy, morals, values and stuff that always seemed important yet eluded so many. Martin Amis would have been proud of him. Ben was classed as a bit eccentric. His simple innocence being misrepresented as often as the sun shines on a summer's day.

He wrote text books for his students to read. He was only twenty-nine years old when he got the job. Young by anybody's standards for a professor. Whilst working towards his qualifications he had been getting some teaching experience as well. Standing in whilst someone was away for a day, or needed a specialist opinion. Ben could project his ideas, but in the same way as Boris Johnson would bumble, Ben would either incite his student's to appreciate him or to do otherwise. Those who digged this got a lot of joy and education from the man. Those who dissed him either left immediately or laughed too hard. That hurt. Ben would shrug it off. He was made of solid stuff.

So how did Ben become involved as Tim's mentor for his training regime? At least that was his aim. Tim consistently delivered the results, the times, the pace, the commitment. Ben would never compete himself, but boy could he add a psychological edge.

They met over a period of time at various Triathlon meets. Tim would win his races regularly, and attract a lot of attention. Ben followed the sport avidly so got excited at the opportunity that this presented. After one race Ben walked up to the winners' enclosure after Tim's victory and suddenly pronounced a volley of intent.

"Tim, I must say something. I would like to be your mentor."
"Why so?" replied Tim.
"I know you so well by now, your coach wants more for you."
"My coach is my business nob-head, now be a good fellow and toddle off" Tim told him harshly.
"My, oh my, that was unexpected. The name's Williams, Ben Williams. I'm a professor at the college. Here's my card, call me when you have spoken to your coach" Ben offered.
"Yeah, whatever old boy, now if you'll excuse me I have business to attend. Thanks anyway!"

That was the first time they ever met together. Not a complete disaster by any means, more an opening. Tim knew deep down that a psychological mentor would be invaluable, especially with his coach's approval. In fact, he secretly rather relished the prospect.

On his way home after the meet, Ben soliloquized: "The plans we make, the things we say and do; sometimes these things are simply just not enough. After all, the map is never the territory. The story about growing up with a perpetual dream, a dream that consistently thrives even if adapted. A man can stand still in a flowing stream, but not in the rivers of man. For to stand still breeds stagnation. Culture rules this earth; film, television, docudramas, sitcoms, art, literature, news, music, poetry, prose, narrative, ways, why's and wherefores." This clarified something in his own mind.

He frequently contemplated all sorts of issues, especially with a moral or philosophic slant to it. These things he lived for.

*

Charlie Morris was simultaneously doing time on a secure ward. He had been sectioned for six months and had picked up an ASBO. He had wanted to set up a small business but his Dad had stopped him. So Charlie attacked his father and smashed a house brick through the front window. Nil support, no sponsorship, no loans, just an angry young man with big ideas….. Charlie knew what he was on with. All he needed were the right finances. He had various passions to follow through with for his business.

Unbeknown to Charlie he was destined to come across Alex Davies when he regained his freedom. He would also meet Claire Halls within a period of two months. Charlie was always adamant, he remained committed to his own cause. He capitalised on his experiences and would go on to meet Ben Williams for the first time as well.

Usually a gentle giant, he worked out a lot at the gym. He generally lived a life of good deeds, he had good karma, positive energy, and many folk would say that they found him to be a friendly and highly practical person to know. He had helped quite a number of people with various projects prior to falling foul. His anger was entirely related to his father's disapproval. Charlie was in a position where he had to prove himself where he felt that that was not necessary. He needed to win faith in himself as much as anything.

By hitting his father, that morph of character caused an alarm to go off within the family. They all said he should be taken away before anything more severe came about. And it could have as well. Charlie was a man with a vision. A man on a mission. He had other ideas where some were happy with none.

Nothing came from nothing. Better to do or have something than nothing at all. His philosophy stemmed from an existential background. Better to have improved what you already had and make a development. The best things would always come to those who prepared. He also knew that the best laid plans of mice and men can gang aft aglay if the wind were to change direction. He knew not to count on the wind staying the same forever.

Although Charlie had qualifications in Economics and Business Studies, he didn't wish to take his studies any further. He just wanted to get his hands on and start-up a business. And he knew exactly what kind of business as well. A tropical fish shop, full of aquaria and marine life for people's living rooms, bedrooms, restaurants, receptions, or wherever else deemed worthwhile.

He was always a determined character. In earlier years he would win his fights and stand-up for the smaller victims that other people picked on. Charlie was admired and respected. A very phlegmatic person all in all.

Basing his projections on personal observations of local and global market forces by reading the *Financial Times, Time* and *Fortune* Magazines, he had decided to commence a designer blueprint for his venture. He began to get flustered with that fact realising that it would take time to come up with. So he needed a network to work with.

What would be the purpose of his store? What value would it add to the society in which he lived? What sense of contribution would he receive for building a new enterprise? Should he go ahead? Was he ready for this? If he got the loan, would he be in a position to repay them within five years as requested?

All these questions and many more came into being for Charlie as he thought about his store to be. Definitely tropical fish though. This was his aim. A local tropical fish shop, called what exactly? This was as yet unknown and would be determined as time went by. He just knew that he could make it work.

However, for the time being Charlie was under supervision, and with no current material freedoms to his name, he felt to be time-rich. Whilst in remand Charlie set about his designer blueprint from the top of his head. It was his good fortune to be transferred to that unit in September. There, he would meet Claire, initially through her music. He had an eye for talent and he knew that whatever shit had just gone on of recent, there was a light to be shone, and that light was Claire Halls.

However, before the two had even met, he had to contend with the authorities of the secure ward who were insistent on giving him medication as long as he was in their jurisdiction. Charlie, in fact, had other ideas regarding the matter.

One day when the senior nurse approached him requesting Charlie to come forwards for 'medication time', Charlie simply said 'No, I won't'. The nurse couldn't believe his ears at this pointed reply. "Now look here Mr Morris, you'll only make things worse for yourself by not complying with us."

"You heard me. I'm not having what I don't need so back off you lousy bastard!" said Charlie.

With that the nurse disappeared into the main office and Charlie was on his way once again.

For two hours nothing much happened, just a glimpse and a stare at him and an occasional turning of heads from through the office window. He opted for a quieter air of indifference during this given timeframe.

He was in his room when it happened. He was minding his own business when five nurses appeared at the door in his room with intent to inject. Charlie detected their intention so got in there first and kicked the first man in the balls and swung his fist into a face before being jumped on and pinned down by four nurses on each arm and leg, and one to administer the injection.

"Fuck off you bastards! You fucking queer pack of rats! Get your hands off me you fat wankers! What the heck do you think you are doing? What gives you the right to lech upon my human rights? You're all a bunch of incompetent cunts – every one of you! Do you have no clue who I am? I am the Champion, and you know it! You bastards - What's in that thing? What's in it?" he screamed at the top of his lungs.

"Haloperidol and Lorazepam" answered a nurse as she administered one injection into each buttock having just fumbled to undo his belt for a moment.

The incident was soon over and left Charlie with an anger, a permanent loathing and disrespect for them. They got up from him cradling their wounds and Charlie just lay there feeling melancholy by what had happened. It totally sucked. The whole game was bullshit. Charlie just had to survive. He had a good mind to throw a table through their window in protest, to make a statement.

As far as they were concerned, Charlie was being given treatment, and as far as he was concerned, he was a businessman looking for an opportunity to further his life and career. He had soon written up the blueprint and that would be enough to go on for the time being. His script had manifest and that would lead him to build from that moment hence.

*

Claire Halls was being resuscitated. She had been beside herself in a creative trough. Feeling rubbished by the world, underappreciated, disrespected and undervalued; having spent the last seven years working on her song-writing skills, she figured that it was time to spare herself from the hassle of even trying anymore. Claire had not accounted on meeting Charlie Morris within three months of that fated summer. Within a year they would be flying on the wings of angels together.

When Charlie first heard her play a good song he would say "it was good." When he heard a great song he would say "it was great." But if he had heard trash he would not have hesitated to say so. When the music he was listening to came from a pure and revolutionary creative force, original sounds resonating forth, words just failed him. In his eyes, Claire Halls happened to write her music from this perspective.

Charlie went into raptures.
"Blows you away sweetheart"
"Cuts to the core"
"Gets you every time"
"Brings emotion where a void once existed"
"Produces the optimism that youth aspires towards."

These were just some of the accolades that she had received from him. Prior to this, she had been desperate. Her own bubble of depression had taken hold of her. No record contract, just the same old grind. "What's the point?" She constantly reflected. Seven years of hard graft on the music front and nothing to show for it except a line of songs that nobody in the sodding pub ever appeared to listen to. "Where's the joy in that?" "Where's the purpose, the sense of valued contribution?" she mused.

In following her heart she had been badly bruised psychologically, owing to lack of interest. No faith. Not even any sign of radical acceptance. Who would ever accept this? She wanted out before she had even taken off.

Her good fortune was to still have Tim as a friend. He still had the magic going on. "Fuck 'em all!" he would frequently utter his famous line during his visits. The message to Claire was to keep going, keep plugging away. She had made this mysterious contact with the outside world, and still had a spark – tiny yes, but present nonetheless. Tim was an old school friend, and had secretly been Claire's No.1 fan. Always appreciated her college gigs although Claire never particularly realised this fact until she was recovering on the ward and suddenly Tim heard the news and appeared to visit from time to time.

So here we had Ben, Tim, Claire, and Charlie all involved together in some way, all looking for something better, some way to find meaning in their lives, and purpose. Perhaps their ideas were much bigger than their actualities. As ever, noone could control the weather. The rain always came once in a while, like it or lump it. Their territory was changing fast.

Claire had an unaccountably dark mood to contend with. She really had tried to end it all. No intentions of carrying on. She was in a rut. No boyfriend, no recording contract, not enough gigs, too much heckling without reckoning for it. She wanted out, so took herself off one morning and did a depressing thing. She was discovered by a man walking his dog. Fortunately, he had a mobile phone on him and the ambulance arrived within fifteen minutes. They had instructed him to put her in the recovery position and check she didn't drown on her own vomit. The man remained anonymous, although there was some gratitude expressed to him.

She could not speak, just articulating mumbles and murmurs whilst her eyeballs rolled back in their sockets. She survived. She did not intend to, hence the deserted field. God knows how long she had been laying there for. Another hour and she would have died for sure.

Her mind had raced and there were images of Charn, the place of cruel sand where all creation crumbled to dust. The place of sad desolation where once, architecture stood aloft. Charn, a place where evil ran rife, the high witch ruling for nothing other than death and misery to the poor wretched within. The cackling beast, whose laughter covered so much beneath. Her nose has grown beyond all sizeable conceit, oh what magnificent deceit.

Plans fell apart, so faltered the here and now. Hope was not lost – "reach deep within your soul and carry on, mistakes in the bag demonstrating what it is to watch everything you gave your life to broken, squeezed, crunched and decimated under your nose. Only the reality is there still, just across the fence, people lived the life in style; The blessed crew embracing life and love as one defined opportunity -love one another." Claire's inner voice told her as she sat thinking.

Charlie met Claire for the first time in the Occupational Therapy Department. They were an instant hit, creative beings, with various aspirations, whether musical or entrepreneurial. Yet to be fully valued and appreciated. Their meetings were restricted to this place as the whole establishment divided the men and women. This made it even more worthwhile when they actually met two or three times a week. Both twenty-somethings, Charlie with his wild enthusiasms for innovation and Claire with her innovative music creations. They were involved in a short space of time. Claire would entertain those attending therapy, the 'troops', with her troubadour skills. Charlie would be also a keen creative artist. He could paint, draw, colour, collage, mosaic, sketch, illustrate, graphically portray any character and so on. He could etch, use chalk, pastels, crayons, pencil, and watercolour. He could be considered the complete artist. His business ideas stemmed from his love of perpetual innovation.

After five weeks worth of meetings, Claire took him to one side whilst the supervisors made tea in the kitchen. "Wanna have some fun?" she asked suggestively.

"What...now? Alright" Charlie quickly replied.

They made their way into a cloakroom and proceeded to embrace, kissing one another, all the while making progressive explorations. This lasted less than five minutes when there was a knock on the door. "Anybody in?" the voice enquired.

"Blast" thought Charlie. They had been rumbled.

Never before had his artwork had quite as much enthusiasm to it as for the next few occasions following that. "So we're going out then?" he asked her when they met.

"I guess so" she said back to him.

"I think Carl knows what happened"

"Oh, really? That's the way the cookie crumbles I guess" she uttered indifferently, not caring about the love bite left on Charlie's neck.

When they got talking they both vowed to set out to make it to the big time immediately upon release. Also, Charlie was able to present and revise his designer blueprint for a tropical fish store. He loved fish and had looked after them as a kid at home. Once he went on holiday to Lanzarote in the Canary Islands and went on a day trip scuba-diving. The fish he saw in that ocean made his imagination explode.

Claire made a pact with him to keep writing her songs until a recording contract came about. 'One a week' became her mission. She told him that she had tried to kill herself because nobody was interested in her or her godforsaken music. The Doctors had tried her on Sertraline, Clozaril and Zyprexa. What she didn't realise was that there would be a new horizon just round the corner.

There would be no hiding the fact that her talent should be shared. With patients, with staff, with Charlie, with visitors, with the world beyond the confines of a hospital ward. Claire had a profound need to have a sense of contribution. This need was not being met so she took an overdose out of sight from her domineering parents. She wanted to, although her music was too good to die like that, and she knew it. Right in the back of her mind she just knew she could offer something to the world. She could contribute. She knew it. But something told her to get out; to leave her misery, and find a happy place. Where the music would always be there, where she would have someone to look after her. She just knew.

This is why she came round again, after all. Her parents and brother looking on with anguish in their hearts. The equipment plugged into her was no cause for alarm, merely a means to survive. Claire was a survivor that time. Even so, she was taken for observation in a hospital. She only wanted her guitar. Apart from that she seemed lost to all. No sense in dithering. That's how she appeared on the ward. Dithering in front of Coronation Street, Emmerdale, Hollyoaks, Brookside, Holby City, Eastenders, not particularly bothered by the activities unfolding before her very eyes. Dithering whilst waiting for tea and toast, dithering while the nurses tried to talk with her. She was not interested. Just in making new sounds, new music. This would occupy her soul. This prospect would be her survival strategy during her time here.

Were it not for Charlie, Christmas on the ward would have been no fun whatsoever. They had put up a tree, decorations, cards, and had even had a Santa come to visit with a sack full of gifts. As people looked on the familiar figure bellowed:

"Ho, ho, ho! Merry Christmas to one and all!"

Nobody responded, even as St Nicholaus gave individual presents he received barely a glimpse of gratitude. Everyone was too far gone. Alison and Michelle, two nurses, came in to cheer everyone on, even started singing 'God rest ye merry gentlemen' and 'Away in a manger' to an antagonised Claire. She figured they were taking the Mickey.

Claire called out to ride Santa's reindeer and was duly disappointed: "they're outside Claire; no, you must stay in now, it's dark outside."

Never before had Christmas seemed so manic. Charlie, being the businessman began to determine and assess the net worth of Santa's sack full of goodies. He reckoned they had been bought from the local shops round the corner, or at least, pushing the boat out, elsewhere in town.

Charlie needed no consolation however. He said 'thankyou' and duly uncovered a triple pack of Reebok sports socks. 'Oh, not bad dude, I can hop, skip, and jump now on my way to the front of the tea queue'. 'No need to be sarcastic now Mr Morris' reprimanded by Chris the evening manager.

With that, Santa vacated the premises and went on his way, presumably back to Lapland for a refill, or more likely to get changed and shaved in time for the New Year. The people of the moment returned to the most challenging and mindless pursuits of telly watching, glazing over and attending to a rumbling stomach by attracting the attention of a passing sexy nurse and demanding toast or snack material.

"Dude, you're surely gonna have yourself a heart attack at that rate, the amount of junk you take in. Try a banana, an apple, a piece of fruit. Those cakes are no good man! Honest, I swear to God, do yourself a favour." Charlie could probably see something else, trying to give someone else a chance at survival.

For the first time, Charlie had heard about Tim and Ben. Claire had recently told him of Tim's last visit. Tim had mentioned that some asshole wanted to be his mentor. No favours expected. Claire nonchalantly uttered 'oh, really?' even though she could not have given a monkey's ass for the matter. Tim kind of felt intrigued that some stranger would want to be a part of his winning machine. Even though, at this stage, there was no impetus. He would still have to speak to his coach first.

Charlie began to assemble some more mental artillery from his conversations. He knew how strong Tim must be judging by his lean physique and track record. He even began to feel a touch jealous that his now girlfriend was being visited regularly by a fan. A fan that had previously been in the background on that particular scene. Tim had quite literally transgressed his usual routine to try and keep her going with the music. He had faith in her songwriting. She was, after all, a born songsmith and people outside of herself could see that. Only, Tim was the first to show it and Charlie knew it too. She needed inspiration, impetus to get that vibe once again properly. Claire required reason, and her reason had been staring her in the face right the way along. It took two close friends to fire it up once again.

The three had been hearing about each other for a while by now. The guys never really actually meeting, even though they both fully knew the score. They knew what was going on. Tim meant nothing more than support. He had a busy training schedule to maintain; why should a suicidal musician stand in his way? No reason, he had decided.

Tim had the most important trials of his entire life coming up within a year. Both focused and a distinct humanist at the same time; a competitive athlete, maybe a philanthropist.

Charlie had the designer blueprint to attend. Thus pursuing his vision, and acquire people on the way. Claire was the first in his hands. She had become a miniature obsession for him. "Must check that girl, she'll pull through – as sure as the waves on the ocean trough, they must come to peak once again. She'll be fine now, I'm sure."

He had always been an optimist through his whole life, even when it got nasty. Charlie had been born with positive blood in his veins. He oozed charisma. Hence the karmic and seismic shift attracting the two together in a heartbeat.

He had no fear actually. Charlie was a brave man. He may have feared his overbearing father as a kid, but the incident had cleared his head of that and now he felt to be the master of his fate, the commander of his ship and destiny. His tropical fish store was calling, his girlfriend was forming musical nuggets, and he had acquired a new indirect friend in Tim.

Tim would, over the forthcoming weeks, mull over the prospect of having a mentor and weighing up the benefits of an improved performance correlating to an improved psychology, or team-building morale. He figured that if this fella who called himself Ben Williams was to be mentor, he would take up the opportunity. After all, he could always fire the guy if it didn't work out.

Time would tell. Charlie wasn't Tim's coach; that was another matter altogether. Maybe Ben was getting ahead of himself here. From fan to Mentor in one fell swoop. Maybe he had a point.

Meanwhile, back in OT, rumours had been circulating about the activities of the two love-birds. They were real enough. Circumstances pending, the two were stuck in a quandary. The least that hope could offer had brought them together to make plans for a brighter future. They began to paint diamonds in the sky, bright lights amongst crochets, quavers and minims. The music would come. Claire had been strumming to herself in the afternoon, she didn't realise the whole room had stopped everything to listen.

They had almost stopped breathing, just holding their breath as her magnificent tones bounced off the walls and struck them where it mattered. That was in their emotional heart. Those who gave a damn appreciated the sounds emitted, otherwise they would listen with a passive interest.

Claire had her hopes renewed now and there was light shining in through the chinks. "Garify the Maripole!" said one abstract comedian to her.

"Thankyou, and you remember to clean between your toes as well", offered Claire for what it was worth.

There were some fairly abstract moments within those four walls at times. Sometimes it could be some TV show, or otherwise someone taking matters into their own hands to get the hell away from the place. Nobody really wanted to end up suffering mass attrition and decomposition by proxy, but the days ticked by and certain things became neglected, whilst some choices were exemplified. Maybe even things that had never really mattered before, until the circumstance presented itself in such a fashion.

Both characters did not particularly like the obligations presented to them. The alternatives, also exhibited, seemed less appealing so Charlie got round to swallowing some pride and getting on with his newfound role there. Claire too found herself adapting to a different environment. She had found purpose, that was the main thing. They were onto something.

Meanwhile, as Tim visited for an hour every weekend he was constantly learning about the goings on of Claire and Charlie. Tim brought in some CD's for her to put on the stereo. He talked about Beijing to her. The Games had massively inspired his training. He felt that he did in fact stand a chance at team selection for London 2012. His results proved to be in good shape, often winning the local races and gaining offers en route of various kinds.

Ben had asked, and the answer was yet to come. Would Tim allow him to be his psychological mentor? After all, what could an Ethics Professor teach an elite athlete about being an elite athlete? That would remain to be seen. Ben felt confident that he could help out in some valuable way.

He had an air of gratitude that Tim would even contemplate his role. Regarding their relationship, this was brand new unchartered territory. Surely Tim would see the light and employ yet another expert to improve his performance. Anything to shine above the others he wished. Surely the magic genie could solve his predicament for him. Ben never claimed to be a magic genie however, but understood that he could help if Tim wanted.

Claire had learnt from Tim about the predicament and subsequently mentioned to Charlie who found the whole thing very funny. He figured that Ben was being a bit too ambitious and should mind his own business, whilst Tim would never choose a mentor over his current coach and club. What Charlie had not figured was that Tim had an open mind and was receptive to suggestion from suitable sources.

This meant that if he sniffed improvement in the air, he would take it on board even if never encountered before. Interestingly for Ben this would mean himself and his methods. "Better to make incremental development than to make detrimental disaster" he thought to himself. On occasion his thoughts leaked out and somebody else got wind of his thinking. Especially when instructing his students. This brought a sense of fulfilment to Benjamin.

Nothing could change the facts about what had happened earlier that year for Claire and Charlie. They would have to face their facts and reevaluate for a while. Whether this would mean triumph or defeat, that was now back in their own hands. They would be back on their feet by 2011 and left to establish a way of life that they could benefit from.

These decisions had already been made within the pair. They would try and try again. "Only mistakes" people agreed. "For surely, were it not for mistakes we would never grow" said a wise person to Claire one day. She agreed and told Charlie next time they met. "Mistakes maketh man", he agreed too.

That wise person was Ben. He had come to meet them through Tim Richardson. Already there were signs of good things to come. As the crew began to form over the months coming, suddenly the world looked to be a different kind of place. No longer just a series of comings and goings, a parade of indifference, a troop of solitary beings; there was something warmer in its place. People coming together to create and fulfil purpose. They reckoned to have found a reason to contribute. Claire had music back, reinstated, and Charlie was able to promote his ideas where it mattered.

Chapter 3
Alex Davies

Alex Davies, who owned the restaurant Collage, had agreed to reserve a table for them all on Thursday evening – the day of Suzanna's birthday. A couple of bands would be playing that night. Folk-rock music, one by a group called Seachimp. Suzanna Jeffries knew Claire Halls, the lead singer, by now as she was dating Charlie, one of Alex's associates.

Alex had always been the entrepreneur, right from an early age, in a similar vein to Charlie. They both successfully collaborated on a kid's comic they invented called 'Squeedge' when still children themselves. The main story was about the battle of the 'Froggle-Bockers' and the 'Mungo-Bubblers'. Alex illustrated and Charlie wrote the stories. They sold each copy for 50 pence from their garden gate.

The other kids, for some reason, loved it and would often save up their pennies to buy a 50p copy of 'Squeedge'. Alex never stopped selling from that moment forth. His eye for venturing had been born. Charlie took great delight in their success at that age. In a typical week they might sell up to 25 copies and split their £12.50 between them both for sweets or extra felt tip pins to draw with. It seemed like a small fortune to the 12 year olds and they felt thus rewarded for their efforts.

Alex's love of food preparation and fine catering began at home, young, as a teenager. He would learn to cook breads, quiches, omelettes and macaroni gratins with his mum– only rapidly expanding into a broader social context meant that his ideas grew too. He knew from the age of fifteen that he wanted to run a café or a restaurant.

To open up his restaurant would have meant years of hard graft. Getting experience from more experienced chefs in pubs, or other hospitality establishments becoming his chief focal point so he dropped out of school at sixteen and began catering college. He was a struggling student as it was, as he suffered dyslexia. The other kids knew this. Oh Lord, how they knew this. They jinxed him in class; unbearably so. He had to get out. His art was good, though. Alex could draw.

By the time he was 23 he had been nominated Head Chef in a local restaurant near Scarborough harbour called 'Ask'. He never gave up his dream to set up on his own sooner rather than later. By the age of 27 he had enough savings and a detailed business proposition to apply for a bank loan and set up his own first business; a restaurant which he decided to call *Collage.* His wife Melanie being something of an artiste, had produced a series of wonderful, bright, colourful mosaics and a couple of collages from famous faces in Hello and OK magazines. Alex took a shine to her artwork and fancied the name to be a winner, so named his restaurant in her honour.

Although *Collage* belonged to Alex, he employed four chefs, and five bar staff/waiters to work the tables at various shifts. His chief mission was success. Alex's objective was to serve the best quality meals at the right price. Nothing got in the way of this for Alex – his life had somehow become one big commitment; commitment to *Collage* and his new family. This was the way of it.

Suzanna, on the other hand, had always wanted to work in a coffee shop but never had the opportunity to do so. She either kept getting refused, or the jobs were simply not available. Her latest application to 'Roasters' coffee shop had been ongoing for three weeks by now, but on account of not being smartly dressed for the interview she doubted her chances of getting the job.

Having already applied to 12 local cafes she began to contemplate Alex. "Would he consider offering me a job here at Collage?" "Would he set up a coffee shop in the future?" "What could I do to get in?"

As it happened, Alex gave her part-time work as a waitress in *Collage.* He had told her of his plans to set up a café as well as the restaurant. All the more because he had the funds available right now. The plan just needed some fine tuning, a name, a property, and the right opening.

Maybe in Scarborough, but ideally in York, she asked what would he call the coffee shop? Alex said that he didn't really know yet, he hadn't thought of that detail, but Suzanna had other ideas:

"The Flaming Squirrels" she suggested.

"Why so?" asked Alex.

Suzanna went on to explain that the name was on account of a vision she encountered on a foreign bus trip. She knew full well that her triathlon training was her physical priority though, so she made no real proposition about the financing of another new business.

"You could train early morning before work,"
suggested Alex.

Suzanna replied "Possibly, although I don't want to
risk burning out."

Alex continued "True comment. True enough. I mean it though; you always were one to stick to your guns."

"Thanks!" she replied enthusiastically.

"You never know, you might catch up with Tim
sometimes?"

"Fat chance of that. Although saying that, I got my
personal best time last week."

"Well done that girl. Excellent performance, really
pleased for you!"

In an aside Alex said to himself "got a best time."

Suzanna carried on: "I'm shy now. Anyway, Tim
is over 20 minutes faster than me and he's on track
for London 2012. More than I can hope for I'm
afraid."

"Your game is on Suzanna. All is not lost. Keep at it!"

The conversation went on for a while, revolving alternatively between business and athletics. They were setting up the restaurant for her birthday meal that evening. Whilst they were busy setting up the tables, there was an air of excitement present, a sense of anticipation as though the evening would be a really good time. Suzanna felt privileged to be working for Alex, especially as he was a stickler for detail and had been known to fire staff for getting things wrong on occasion.

Alex actually had no qualms with Suzanna. He had interviewed her with his wife Melanie and both had agreed to offer her a 3 month trial placement. She had sailed through this period without so much as a glitch and now she was being rewarded with a birthday in the restaurant as part of the 'family'.

They knew full well that all seven of the 'crew' would be present in the evening. Only, Suzanna also felt concerned about her brother; her dearly beloved temperamental brother. Sometimes his mood could go off at a tangent. An unforeseeable, intangible change of mood could make him become aggressive. Sometimes for no good, or no substantiated reason whatsoever. Yes, her brother worried her. Although she did credit him for keeping up the training scheme, as agreed, with Tim. Maybe Shane was envious of Tim. Shane would never get on to Team GB. Tim just might.

Shane was something of a scientist. A potential teacher if only he could control his moods. He needed to get a grip. His knowledge of Physics was beyond elementary. In fact, rather more – way beyond elementary. Shane would entertain the notion that one day, before he reached the age of sixty, he would win the Nobel prize for Physics. This seemed like a long shot in view of his current situation. His circumstance would pit him against the odds. Crikey, there are people who have won the Nobel prize who wouldn't have dared even imagine they would. Their genius exemplified, they did.

Shane Jeffries was a dreamer, but with problems attached. Science could be a dangerous game. People got damaged, animals got tortured, plants got destroyed; all in the name of advancing science.

Shane found that he would get worked up about experiments gone wrong.

Anyhow, he was invited to his sister's birthday at Collage on the Thursday evening. He had determined to ignore Ben Williams though. Maybe a grudge about his perceived sexuality. No one knew for sure though. Ben meant no harm. He was extremely intelligent and had been eventually accepted by Tim as his psychological mentor for training sessions.

Charlie would be there, of course, to offer support to Claire. She had been invited to sing with her band *Seachimp*, by request and arrangement. They usually played some folk-rock numbers and everyone was looking forwards to the musical interlude that evening. Their songs would be valued at least.

That evening, Tim kept fairly quiet the whole time, and Shane too. There was no accounting for Ben's contribution to the evening, as he decided to interject with words of what he perceived to be wisdom as often as possible, but not so much as to detract from the evening belonging to Suzanna, the birthday girl.

Nobody else minded Ben. He was new to the area, and had been granted a position as Ethics Professor on campus. Tim had, after some humming and hawing, accepted him on his coaching plan. Ben was a psychological mentor to him. But his academic nature was sometimes hard to follow.

During the course of the evening people gradually arrived between 7pm and 7.30pm as arranged. Suzanna had been home to change out of her working attire and into something more comfortable for the evening ahead. They would be up for a long time. Probably into the early hours. Knowing Alex, he would shut up shop with the party still indoors. Anyhow, no worries about being kicked out tonight.

It felt great to be waited upon for a change, instead of doing the waiting. They had a mixture of garlic bread, olives, pitta bread, humous, and breaded mushrooms with garlic dip for starters. They all shared these out amongst the group. After a moment, Ben got talking with Suzanna. He was perfectly aware of her ambitions athletically, so tried to tailor his banter to this. He did in fact have a soft spot for her. Would anything come of it? Some people doubted his orientation on account of coming from the outside. Ben was the newest addition to the group. But by no means unpopular.

He blurted out in an attempt to get through to her: "Discipline learnt from the triathlon training could be redirected into setting up your cafe when the time came. Energy to work with and be an entrepreneur would be exponentially connected to competitive athletics in a similar vein to that which you already do."

Tim overheard this statement and guffawed out loud at that. He guessed what it would mean to her to help run a coffee shop/sandwich bar. Besides he rather liked the name she had conjured up. An original concept which would surely hit the spot, so long as all else fell into place.

In the mean time, all Suzanna wanted was to be able to consistently beat her personal best time at Triathlon (which she was doing admirably already), and then, within a 3 year period of time to open up *The Flaming Squirrels* café/sandwich bar and work for Alex. Suzanna was a family friend of the Davies and Melanie knew that this was an accepted and respected fact. There was to be no extra-marital affair going on. Anything of that nature would probably have disbanded her from the set-up.

Suzanna had no objection to Ben's attentions. They made her feel more human if anything. But she couldn't see any further developments with him. Her athletic and business goals were more important at this moment in time. She was a strong-minded woman with a high set of values in her life. She was value-driven. Ben was, too, come to that. Being an Ethics professor, he would frequently contemplate life from a moralistic stance. He was hoping for a wife and family now that he had begun to be established at the University. Understandably so; after all, he had worked so hard to get this far already. Maybe his sensitive disposition made people think twice.

Collage was theirs tonight. The bar would stay open and the time was right. Claire reminded everyone and announced that it was her friend's birthday. To celebrate that fact she announced that the free drinks were there for a cultured toast so she proposed to the world:

"Suzanna… Cheers! Salud! Salut! Prost! Skol!"

Glasses chinked at the table.

"Yes, for all those who didn't know, that was English, Spanish, French, German and Norwegian all in one!" Claire continued. She had been through her difficult patch, an early mid-life crisis. Now she was getting back into the swing of things once again.

Back on her feet once again, and being a bumptious character she was in the band: 'Singer-songwriter, lead figure, multi-lingual and a talented guitarist.' Many people would come to appreciate her music. Thanks to Charlie Morris she had risen, like a Phoenix from the flames and regained a life worth living. There was always going to be a way for her. It had just required somebody to point it out to her. There was a way and that was music. Charlie Morris and music were to be the way for Claire Halls.

Ben then made a promise to learn more languages, himself, to impress his students with. It could add a cultural context to the ethics that he already taught. Although he had never travelled beyond Europe, Ben knew a few words of Mandarin Chinese, and he already knew Esperanto. Ben figured that it made sense to be able to communicate with anybody around the world by means of a universal language. He had not shared this thought with the others yet, though.

Within half an hour, the main courses turned up. There was an excited gasp of exhilaration as the food appeared. There was a selection of meats, vegetables, salads, vegetarian stuff, and it would all be catered for on the bar tab. Suzanna didn't have to pay a penny tonight. Shane would see to it. And with that fact, the whole table would see to it for her.   Charlie had opted for steak (rare), chips, onion rings, peas and French mustard. Claire had gone for a vegetarian Caesar salad with extra croutons. She drank orange juice whereas Charlie opted for a glass of Merlot.

Shane and Suzanna both surprised themselves, going for rack of lamb, minted potatoes, carrots, green beans and shared a bottle of Chardonnay between them. Ben joined them for the Chardonnay despite the evil eye he would get from Shane. Ben fancied breaded chicken with chips, ketchup, peas and salad.

Alex was on duty cooking in the kitchen. He would join them once the restaurant had stopped serving. He had agreed to provide one round on the house and a free birthday dessert for Suzanna, although this wasn't known at the time. He had made special care to pep the food to its peak on this night. Fearing the wrath of Gordon Ramsey, any false moves from his staff would spell serious trouble on this occasion. As it would on any occasion, only he had made it sound more serious for effect.

Tim was content to eat salmon with lemon and dill, boiled potatoes, peas and salad. He drank apple juice as he was teetotalling because of his triathlon commitments. He kept a detailed log of everything that he ate. All proteins, carbohydrates, fats, vitamins, fibres, sugars carefully scrutinized day by day, week by week. His coach was proud of him. Tim had the greatest potential. Who knows, maybe he would qualify for the London Games of 2012. He had the legs. He had the support. He had the speed. He could run like a Cheetah when it came to it.

Their meal was long and drawn out. All were having a good time at the table. Even the more reticent. It got to a point where potatoes and chips were being launched as projectiles across the restaurant. Much to everyone's humour a chip had landed in the glass of another customer. He figured they were having a party, so threw it right back at them hitting Shane square in the face. A soggy chip. Everyone howled with mirth. No apologies necessary.

It came to the time for dessert. A huge gateau had been prepared with strawberries, cream, chocolate chips and candles with an iced message 'Happy Birthday Suzanna'. The waiters sang and John came out of the kitchen especially for the event. Everybody took a slice of the cake, including Tim (rather more reluctantly) and ate it. "Yum!" "Delicious"!

Charlie began to return the compliment to their host and sang "For he's a jolly good fellow" to Alex. Ben and co joined in as well. They were having a merry time.

Seachimp were due to begin playing at 9pm for a couple of hours. After that was anyone's guess.

Once the meal proceedings had been completed, Claire excused herself from the table and set up on the raised stage area to perform. The other band members had arrived and were enjoying a drink at the bar. They got themselves sorted and then the band kicked off; Seachimp began to perform folk-rock. All seven people were there that night. They were the 'crew': Tim, Charlie, Claire, Ben, Shane, Suzanna and Alex.

Tim sat around quietly with Shane in the background. Although it was his sister's birthday, Shane had had precious little to contribute to the conversation. He hated Ben's guts as Ben was about to find out over the next few weeks. He knew already, although not to the extent of what was to come. Shane was convinced that Ben had homoerotic tendencies. It was only Shane who had any malevolent feelings about the man. Nobody else had either a niggle or a complaint.

Ben had no such predisposition. As a matter of fact, he fancied Shane's sister. Suzanna guessed this. The problem was that she fancied Tim so would be unable to return any unrequited love or affection for her. Ben was a patient man. He had waited 29 years to get his first job, why hurry and mess it all up over a woman.

As the band played on into the night, Charlie looked on with pride in his eyes; a sense of personal triumph. Since he had met Claire, between then and now, there had been so much water under the bridge. She had come back from being down to an extreme point in her life and now to being an active songsmith and something of a public treasure. At least, locally anyhow. As far as Alex Davies and Collage were concerned, Seachimp were the house band, even before the recording contract. They would now undoubtedly move onto bigger and better things.

Her singing was captivating, capturing all the pain, anguish, and trauma of a troubled soul perfectly. Claire Halls could move an audience magically. Her emotions took a grip and in the light of what she had been through since this time last year, a tear welled up in Charlie's eyes. Only transitorily, mind.

They took a respite at 11pm and asked if they had had enough yet. "We want more!" they yelled in response. They wanted more, but would have to wait. The band had been playing full out for two hours straight by now. She needed a break, a breather.

And a breather they all got. Alex had agreed to let them stay on until the early hours in the restaurant. Ben was alluding towards Suzanna all night, much to Shane's disgust. She never took offence at this, at least not visibly. Ben was a determined character and would never be the first to give in on a mission when it came to that.

Alex had cleared up the kitchen and came to join the party. "Well, well, well, what a to-do," he declared. "This was worth a night off work, hey Suze."

"Thankyou so much, I really appreciate what you guys have put on for me", she replied.

"You'll have to have a birthday more often", mentioned Charlie.

"Yeah, and Claire will have to perform more often as well. Lest we forget, we've just been entertained by the world's finest. The one and the only, the no-longer-up-and-coming-more-made-to-the-core 'Seachimp'!" announced Ben.

"Top stuff guys. You're a cool dude, Ben; hope you get your dog soon" Claire contributed.

For in truth, Ben had plans to acquire a canine companion to keep him company. Man's best friend and all that. Nothing had occurred as of yet, but he figured that within a five month period there would be some action taken on this notion. For some reason, he must have mentioned it in passing, but the crew seemed to understand his ideas as far as this was going anyhow. Probably a proper dog; a Dalmatian, a Spaniel, a Collie, a Labrador, a Pointer, or a Whippet.

He wouldn't be tempted to go for a Jack Russell, or a Terrier type tiddler. Alex had specified that Collage would not allow animals in the premises. This would be understood.

He had recently sacked somebody for dropping and smashing dishes three times in one week. He wouldn't stand for carelessness, especially when the warnings had been stated perfectly clearly in the first instance. Alex was a man of his word. So was Charlie come to that. This is probably why they got on so well. They had a mutual understanding. They were childhood buddies, and as fortune would have it, they remained in contact into their twenties, through thick and thin, as entrepreneurs.

Melanie was beautiful, intelligent and loyal to Alex. She was independent, but chose to help around Collage as a business partner in her own right. Nothing would please Alex more than a good day's work in the restaurant. He would often go out on excursions to look for more suppliers. He believed in serving quality meals at the right price. Therefore, he sometimes took the weekend to travel up north, or to the Midlands, in search of new recipes, fine cuisine, fresh ingredients and authentic chefs to validate the menu.

Melanie had suggested travelling abroad to get the best alternatives. "The French would teach you a thing or two" she said. "They are known for their haute cuisine n'est-ce pas?".

"Yes, I would like to explore some continental recipes, as well as some Indian Spice and Mediterranean fish dishes. The Greeks have a very healthy diet and we could go on holiday for a week to explore the possibilities," Alex replied.

They certainly would have their work cut out for them over the years, especially with a steady staff at hand, plenty of folk looking to get in on the act and a potential coffee shop/sandwich bar just round the corner. The funds were all in place by now and Alex would have to make the right approaches at the right times. He mentioned already that his chief waitress would be welcome to work as a barista. Suzanna felt this opportunity would be most welcomed so was on edge about the move.

Alex's dyslexia wasn't something that people made judgement of. However, it meant that he couldn't read or write very well. So, with that in mind he would hire his staff to write out the menus, to type up the business plans, the blueprints, and usually, if it came to the time of signing a leasing contract, he would have Melanie by his side to ensure that no small print would do him out of business. She was a smart cookie.

Collage was a small business; a thriving small business. Everybody knew each other's dealings within the restaurant and consequently, it could be said that there was an atmosphere of trust and respect within. Alex figured that any business lacking in trust would go bust within a very short period of time. In fact, if somebody broke his trust, or crossed him in any way, they would probably be fired without too much of a to-do.

His was a method of constant improvement. The Japanese called it 'Kaizen', the Americans called it 'CANI™' (Constant And Never-ending Improvement). Alex just called it hard work. He would be there early mornings until late at night to see his business functioning properly. Alex Davies was a man of integrity. He enjoyed seeing his ideas flourish and would be sad to see his hard work go wrong.

Once in a while there would be trouble with a customer. Maybe a complaint about the food or something, maybe a chair was uncomfortable, perhaps the table wasn't big enough for a group of diners. Or it could be that the drinks were considered to be too expensive, even though they were set at a standard rate according to national price regulation.

However, for the main part of its existence, Collage was a fairly synchronised business. Clients would come and go feeling satisfied about the quality they had received. To begin with Alex would leave feedback forms on the tables in order to learn what could be improved in the establishment. Not everyone filled out these forms though.

Alex and Melanie were a star item in the local community. Now that they had family, they would soon have to consider schooling as well. They both agreed that local schools would provide the best opportunites for Fiona. Although they could probably afford private schools, Alex figured that he would rather she grew up to understand the world of hospitality from an early age. That may have seemed ambitious, but that was the way that they had decided to grow it forwards. To pay it forwards would mean a stronger bond, a more together family unity. Thus, a fully functioning Davies' enterprise would exist. Alex had big ideals really. Only time would tell.

Melanie would campaign once a year for the Green party. She was an environmentalist. She believed in recycling, and sponsoring Greenpeace. She would often buy products from The Body Shop, and even considered buying an acre of rainforest to prevent deforestation in Indonesia, or South/Central America. She was a good egg. Alex had done well by her at his side. It took two to tango and these two could salsa, baby!

Being an artist, Melanie had applied to the National Music and Arts Council for a grant to enable her to complete some further works of art. They had been impressed by the set-up and a representative actually came to visit and held an interview on the premises of Collage. She had been granted £1500 to buy canvases and materials, and what's more, had gained a new clientele. They would come back with other people further down the line to inspect the finished works and to provide an estimate about values, etc.

The artist within admired the solid rock that Alex made out to be. He was a rock of empathy, a solid Great Oak through storm, wind and weather. They hadn't always had the same affinity. For instance, in the early days she had merely been a customer visiting with an old boyfriend. She discovered his bachelor status and understood the potential that could lay within the man. She swooped and scored. Yeah man, Alex didn't stand a chance, once he was in her sights that was it. Soon he came round to the idea and pulled out all his stops. They were definitely a coup for the Scarborough community.

Alex had a good local knowledge too. If somebody asked what was on in town, he would know at least three or four events or places worth going to that same day, every day. Collage provided a 'what's on guide' in the foyer, so curious folk could find out for themselves where to go during the week.

The restaurant was no minor undertaking though, even though classed as a small business, it demanded full-time attention. Alex would often be up before 6am to ensure there were enough provisions for the day, to check the kitchen was in order, the cutlery all present, the crockery ready for the new day. He was an early riser and a short sleeper. A real hard-worker, and always had been since the age of 19. Having left school with just a handful of GCSEs that he had scraped through by some minor miracle, the odds were certainly stacked against him in the line of catering. Some folk had years on him. He was, at first, treated like a dog's body in the industry. Within five years he had turned this round and had begun to lead the proceedings.

Whilst he worked at 'Ask' he had learned many useful aspects of catering. He had saved up hard, worked harder, and developed a blueprint for Collage. There were a couple of co-workers who had expressed an interest to work with him in his new line of business. Being a seaside, Spa and fishing town, there were plenty of opportunities for maritime activity, although within the town there seemed to be a battle going on between the fishermen and the townsfolk. Who owned the territory? Whose turf were they on exactly? Alex had the good fortune to be a talented chef. He had become accepted over the years, to the point of which he could both afford to and had the know-how to run a business.

Alex Davies was a cool guy. Like Charlie Morris, he had ideas, he had a vision, and he had a reality. They both understood the bounds, the territory, the whys and wherefores of organisational proceedings. Alex was married, Charlie had saved Claire's life. She had been down and as good as out when they met. But that was now by the by in another time and place. Alex had more status and was better founded, but Charlie was not merely the upstart either. He could write his own blueprints, he could even advise on what to include. Alex would consult with him on occasion.

Although considered a cool guy, Alex wouldn't exactly aim to be the winner of a popularity contest. He had principles and would stick to them, to the extent of argument if deemed necessary. He would frequently win at these too, as he had many years' experience. Melanie was not ashamed to open up fully with points or issues raised either for or against. Sometimes it may make Fiona uncomfortable seeing her parents rally like this. Most often, the air would clear very quickly after a discussion.

Alex had always dreamed of running a restaurant since around the age of fifteen. He had learned his basic skills at home with his mum. She had provided the items and he had gone at it with vigour. His energy had never died down since those days. A rapid rise to employment from leaving school had given him the chance and the opportunity to avenge his demons. Although not a religious man, Alex would attend to Collage with almost religious attention. Extremely fastidious would be a better word for him.

He was atheistic in background. A business person, the same as Charlie, he devoted his time to the task at hand. He was dedicated and committed. Set in his ways, but adaptable when the time came. Alex Davies was extraordinary. He had the advantage of experience in years. Collage had proved a roaring success and there were no indications that this small business would flounder. His goal was expansion, extending his proprietorship to the café within three years. Already, Suzanna was eagerly anticipating working there. It would mean a livelihood on top of training. She had reached her physical peak and it was now a matter of maintenance.

She thoroughly enjoyed the early morning swims at the local pool with Tim and co. But the commitment was enormous. She would, on occasion, come home quite fatigued, so much so that the rest of the day was a difficulty. She never admitted this to anyone because she wanted to be brave. She wanted to be responsible for Tim's place on Team GB and to get him to the London Games on time.

Somedays Tim would just leave Sainsbury's and get out his BMX. He was still a teenager at heart, and loved nothing more than impressing the fans with super-cool-stunts. He could pull them all by now. Had been practising since the age of twelve. Read all the magazines, been to the parks, hung out with the right crowd, broken his arm twice in the process, and was the proud owner of a Diamondback BMX bike on top of his Trek Madone triathlon bike. Tim, in fact, relied on Suzanna to motivate him at that hour on a morning. She was a key player for him. To lose her now would be a disaster.

Even though she fancied him, as she was so avidly hiding from him, she was bursting. And still in Collage on her birthday she was caught between Ben's attentions, Shane's animosity, and reaching out for Tim. To do so may end their training partnership. This would be a major event.

So much so, that there were no actions taken in Collage on that night. The crew stayed until 2am, then, by mutual consensus they decided to leave. Alex attempted to play a few chords on guitar for them all, but his forte lay with hospitality. They agreed that the music should be left to Claire. She took extra delight in this. And Charlie made an expression as if to say 'I knew this all along!'

The birthday had been a great event. Everybody had played their part. Collage had been thriving that night. The rounds had been coming in, and the food was good. Seachimp were due to return there within a fortnight; so they felt satisfied and collected a wage from Alex. He had made a 15% discount on the overall tab as well, as a gesture of goodwill. Nobody complained about this.

Charlie went home with Claire, Shane and Suzanna went back to their parent's home 20 minutes walk away, Ben caught a taxi to the top of town, Tim thanked Alex for a fantastic time, and Alex shut up shop ready for a new day.

He was there with Melanie just thinking about that night. They felt happy and appeased that the proceedings had been straightforward as planned. Both wanted to say something but could think of nothing. So they embraced instead. The embrace lead to a kiss on the lips and they looked into each others eyes meaningfully for a lingering moment.

It was getting late now and the restaurant was shut for the night. Everyone else had gone, Fiona was long since asleep and they were buzzing from the evening's events. Melanie looked at Alex suggestively as they stood in the kitchen. He smiled, acknowledging her intent. They had another hug, this time a little harder and with hands exploring body parts.

They both simultaneously sighed a breath of pleasure and proceeded to kiss more passionately, tongues and manipulating each others heads in a physical way. Alex coaxed Melanie to sit on the main table in the middle of the room whilst he pressed himself close up between her legs. She moaned with relief. He proceeded to caress her thighs and sides whilst she placed her right hand onto his crotch and squeezed teasingly.

Alex suddenly gushed with hot blood as the mood altered from end of night to raw sex. He ripped off her jumper and cupped her peaked breasts in both hands. She returned fire and removed his shirt in a flourish. Shoes came off fast and Alex discovered his trouser belt presented no problem to a highly skilled Melanie. By now he was fully erect and aroused and she was urging his fingers into her warm, moist mound. This movement caused them to forget themselves and they were both lost in passion.

As she bent over the kitchen table she urged him to plunge his monument deep inside her and they gyrated for quite some time together before a climactic groan came from Alex and a satisfied, mischievous sound erupted from Melanie. They were both spent for the night now and collapsed on the table for five minutes still naked.

"We'd better put your chopper away, don't want to mix the meat and veg up for tomorrow do we Alex", gasped Melanie as they grinned together looking up at the ceiling.

"Come on then, we'd better go up for the night. Early start again tomorrow hun", Alex replied.

With that they got partially dressed once again and made their way to the domestic quarters for a night's sleep, content in the knowledge that they were fulfilled once again.

Chapter 4
Sibling Rivalry

The month of April 2011 had arrived. Shane and Suzanna Jeffries had both been accepted to run the London marathon. On a charity placement, they had pledged to raise £3,000 for Macmillan's Cancer Research between the two of them. An Aunt had died of cancer some years previously, and so they were both left with a sense of duty to actively further research into the area. They had been left with a sense of loss, but had come to terms with it over the years since then.

Although the triathlon would be their preferred sport, there were implications for greater things if they could cover a marathon first. Both had their eyes on a sub-3hour run, although would be happy to complete the course at all. There would be a whole team for Macmillans. In a way, it seemed a shame not to be running for The Blue Cross instead, as she loved animals, but the cause was understood and a positive fund came from their targeted sponsors.

They had been training over progressive distances since August time the previous year. By November they were up to a half marathon standard, completing a couple of local events to confirm their fitness. Shane had the upper hand on his sister, beating her time by a good amount. He was multi-talented, being able to swim, cycle and run. And what is more, he had a black belt in Taekwondo, too. He had studied the martial art since the age of twelve with the WTF school (World Taekwondo Federation). There were three main schools in the UK, TAGB (Taekwondo Association of Great Britain), ITF (International Taekwondo Federation) and WTF – Shane's arena.

He had aggressive tendencies, but athletics helped him channel his energies into something constructive. Being competitive he felt the need to win if at all possible. He got a malicious sense of satisfaction at being faster than his sister. He was also her protector. He would stand in if any untoward outsider were to come forwards. He often would let her and the world know that he was looking out for her.

During his teenage years Shane would attend Taekwondo meetings and tournaments. He had become exceptionally fit. He was in good shape, young, flexible, strong, and had Suzanna's trust. He would get upset when intrusions were made upon their sibling relationship; jealous in a way. With the exception of training with Tim, Shane and Suzanna were a bit of a clique. At home they would produce detailed notes and training schedules. Even their daily nutrition was precisely recorded: Calories, Proteins, Fats, Sugars, Carbohydrates, Vitamins, Minerals, and Fibre etc. Shane kept a chart on a kitchen cupboard with all the week's nutrition checked on a regular basis.

His mum would sometimes joke about his anal behaviour. Finding it to be too pernickety or something, she would insinuate that he needn't be such a stickler for dietary observations, so long as he would eat properly every day – a light breakfast, or porridge in the winter for its carbohydrate content. He would often settle for fruit in the morning – all morning – and then a salad lunch with carbohydrate, and a protein meal in the evening. Knowing where he was with his specific diet gave him an edge, as well. He feared obesity, and felt emotional about the prospect of ever becoming fat himself. He would hate to lose his form owing to careless diet planning. That would go down as a personal nightmare for Shane. He feared very little, but that would be one thing he couldn't bear to think about.

Suzanna, on the other hand, would often go all out with high carbohydrate content pasta meals. She could pile a plate up high with spaghetti, or twirls, or some other pasta content and scoff the lot. She trained hard, and had her brother to keep her on track if necessary. They never went too far wrong with each other's guidance. Subscribing to 'Runner's World' and 'Triathlon 220' magazines provided the necessary education for maximising their potential on the course. There had been a three month countdown to the marathon itself, beginning in January. Distance to be increased – one long Sunday run and the rest of the week fartlek, intervals, strides, swimming, cycling, or an alternative such as squash in the gym centre.

Sometimes Shane would play Tim just recreationally on a morning. There was very little to separate the scores between these two contenders. On the triathlon course Tim would win hands down, but on a squash court there was more fair game to be had. Shane was fit. Tim was fit. Providing there were no injuries, the training would continue and the courses would be completed.

Back on the marathon, the time had come. It was April 2011. The two siblings were prepared and now entirely prepped up for the event. The run was due to commence early at 8.45 am from Greenwich Park. This had meant a super early 5 am start when Shane and Suzanna completed a full stretching programme and included half an hour's yoga. They had come to London two days earlier and were staying in hotel accommodation. Aiming to arrive at the start line for 8am, they ate breakfast at 6.30am – porridge and a croissant with orange juice. Both had a banana for the start line and a bottle of lucozade sport.

They were surrounded by 30,000 participants, all coming together for this common cause. Hundreds of charities were represented , people dressed up in costumes ranging from a tin of Heinz baked beans to Sponge Bob, to the crowd of soldiers on the march with backpacks on, from Transvestites to Wedding Belles, from Mr Blobby to Superman. All possible representations were on that course; many, like Shane and Suzanna, wearing a more conservative charity vest with shorts and running shoes. Shane wore Asics Cumulus trainers, and Suzanna wore New Balance. There were thousands of pumped up people present that morning. This was a big event.

They would run past the renovated Cutty Sark, repaired from the 2007 burns. They would run across Tower Bridge, and through the streets of London town for 26.2miles (42km). As fortune would have it they were ready.

As they ran they split up but kept up a familiar pace. They had arranged to meet up at the end at the meeting place beginning with 'J'…..'J for Jeffries'.

What an incredible achievement! Shane came home in 2hrs 52 minutes, and Suzanna made it in 3hrs 10minutes. Maybe not as fast as would have been liked, but a complete, injury free circuit nonetheless. They received a medal, t-shirt and refreshment bag of goodies to recover with.

As arranged they met at the 'J' sign and embraced enthusiastically. They were chuffed to bits, all the training had paid off now and they had actually achieved their targets both in sponsorship and in distance. Now all that remained was for the money to be collected and sent to Macmillans. Tim was somewhere in the crowd. He had come to watch the event, and even though they may not have seen him, they appreciated his support, and figured that tit-for-tat they would be there for him too.

With the April marathon complete, it would be back to triathlon territory. A Northern Ripon event would occur in July 2011, following which there would be an August return to London to complete the London Triathlon. Tim would be aiming for a top result in the event. The siblings would train with him between now and then. They were a team – unofficially - but they were understood. The difference between the Jeffries' and Tim Richardson was the quality shown by the results they were pulling in. Tim was Team GB material, Shane and Suzanna were both County material. They competed for North Yorkshire.

At times, however, some real bullshit would often occur with Shane and his training. His father was not fully in agreement with his training and his mother would sometimes ridicule him. They were convinced of their superiority on account of being parents. Not that they would have ever achieved at County level themselves, but they were full of "blah, blah, blah". A talking point with the neighbours perhaps, or a nod and a wink as they learnt of another contest or event. They were full of ridicule, believing Shane's antics to be nonsensical. Although they may, from time to time, buy a pair of trainers, or shorts, or gels, or headwear for him, they never really got into the idea of being there for him at the events. They couldn't see the point.

With Suzanna it was the same. That is why the two siblings got along together to train, and with Tim. Shane had been at school with Tim; they had been in different years, but during the North Yorkshire meets where Tim had won, they had begun to formulate a friendship in training there.

Between April and July time, they had over two full months and a half to train. This would involve early mornings at the swimming pool, or out on the bikes, Tim, Shane and Suzanna pushing themselves to new limits. Every day they would set a target. Whether it was just one second or one metre in improvements they would aim to achieve this goal. Unlike Shane and Suzanna, Tim had a lot more backing behind him. His parents bought him bikes, and would frequently attend the meetings too to show support. Shane and Suzanna were there for him 24/7 and they figured that this was for the best.

It came to July time and the meeting at Ripon. Tim won the race as anticipated, and the two others got good times, keeping their places on the County team. Tim collected a prize for first place, a cheque for £250 and a media article in the local gazette the next morning. He was on track for London 2012 and the whole set-up was looking more and more likely the whole way through.

Like a crusader riding through the night, gallantly by sturdy steed, on horseback strong, Tim would be a favourite. As far as he was concerned, he was up there with the best, the very essence of triathlon; his coach would be there through thick and thin. The results were coming in. The prospect of injury did occur from time to time, but being cut short never really scared Tim. He was too focused. The two siblings helped enormously with this one.

One month later, August came round and it was time for the London Triathlon. The three of them drove to London with the coach and Tim's parents. They were due to check into a Docklands Hotel for a couple of nights and be up early in the morning for the start of the event. They had the trailer with the bikes on for the cycling component of the race. Parking in the hotel car park, they made their way to the check-in.

They moved towards the reception with the bags and checked in for the first night. It was Saturday, and the race was first thing Sunday morning. They had an early night and were in three rooms; Tim and Shane, Suzanna on her own, and Mr and Mrs Richardson. It seemed to be the most convenient arrangement this time round.

Arising at 5am the athletes went through the motions of their stretch and warm-up routines, thus preparing for the day ahead. After they were done they made their way downstairs to have breakfast. Then the three athletes made their way to the start line whilst Tim's parents made their way to a convenient spot from which to offer support.

Standing at the water's edge Tim had his hopes on another big result. He wanted to win this, and he wanted it badly. The training had brought him up to speed as far as this moment, the companionship and partnership with the Jeffries' had enabled him to feel included all along, not withstanding those sole moments of pounding round a track, or pedalling up those inclines reliant on looking deep within. Anyway, the time had come. Could he pull in a bona fide result from this summer event? Or would he be unable to equal his expectations? Only the next two hours would tell!

The starter's claxon sounded and the swimmers were in the water; Tim making a strong start, Shane hot on his heels. At least 150 participants were taking part in this Olympic distance race. They would have to swim 1.5km, then cycle 40km following which a final 10km run would separate the wheat from the chaff, the men from the boys, the contenders from the also-rans. With a bit of luck, the wind would be good today and blow a nice tidy gust in his sails. The swim was going well. All they had to do was aim for the bouys and avoid being struck by another swimmer's feet or arms as they jet-propelled through the water.

It was over before you could say your 'ABC', the first swimmers had reached the landing stage and were already making their way through the transition. Off with the goggles and caps and wetsuits, on with the trainers and onto the bikes. Off they would pedal along like fury, as though their lives depended on this. For some, yes, their entire athletic career lay in jeopardy at the whims of getting a good result here. For the likes of Tim, he was being closely scrutinised for Team GB potential and the pressure was on. Shane was fit, and required a decent time but without trying to win or even make the top 10. He would be happy with a best time for himself and maintenance of condition, of course.

Suzanna, on the other hand, was entered in the Sprint distance event. That would mean swimming for 750m, cycling 20km, and running 5km at the end; a shorter course in all, but perfectly adequate for her to participate in. She was always on a mission to achieve a new personal best time. Whether this was by the width of a cat's whisker, or the breadth of a freckle on a forearm, she would be content to see an improvement of some description, anyhow.

The race was on, and there was adrenaline pumping everywhere. They were young, fit and courageous. Mr and Mrs Richardson were standing half way round the cycle route yelling, clapping, hopping and encouraging the athletes as they cantered by. Tim was in 7th position after 15km on his bike, having been just in the top 10 after the swim. Shane was much further down the field. Not struggling mind, but just not as fast as some.

The race continued and by the time of the run Tim had gained some ground and was in 5th position. In truth, anywhere in the top 10 was good enough, but being entirely competitive he wanted to win the whole thing and get more credit for it. He valued the status that came with winning and receiving favourable attentions. His coach would be happy with that, and it would keep the ball rolling along the way.

Shane nearly came off his bike at one point; a sharp corner had meant a sudden brakeage to be applied and he miscalculated slightly as he went round. But he kept his balance and continued with the route. He was in the 80's position-wise but he had his eyes on the timer rather than overtaking every man that presented himself en route. There were some wonderful characters doing the event in many shapes and sizes.

By the time the race had ended, Tim had run himself into 4th position and his time was suitable for note. He was briefly exhausted from his exertions but recovered within a 10 minute period. They say that fitness is in the length of time it takes you to recover. He was very fit indeed and toned perfectly in mind, and body. Shane came home in good time unharmed by the days exercise, and Suzanna, too, had had a good run. She knocked off 2minutes 45seconds from her previous pb at that distance. So, a good run and a superb achievement from the three colleagues.

Mr and Mrs Richardson came back to talk with them in the reception arena, and they warmed down and drank some Lucozade Sport to rejuvenate their muscles and get the necessary fluid back into their bodies. Full of sugars and minerals, this drink would be the option for many an athlete during such an event.

"Like lightning, greased lightning, so fast it's not even frightening", sang the three in the car on the way home. Much to their relief the event had been a success, Tim had got noticed favourably, and there were no injuries amongst them. Maybe beginning to feel a little more selfish by now, each had an individual objective in mind for future reference. Tim would be guaranteed a place on the London squad from his recent performances, and the two siblings were touched with empathy and a little envy at the same time.

So the summer of 2011 was still upon them. They all made plans and continued to look ahead again. Shane had decided to run another marathon in the autumn season. He had entered the Amsterdam marathon due to take place at the beginning of October. Nobody else would be with him, just Shane at the event with the other thousands of athletes. Suzanna thought he was a bit mad for wanting to run twice in one year. His parents thought he was out of hand for running marathons at all. They were not happy about this.

But Shane was determined. He would go ahead with the event and train accordingly. Having run the London marathon in April he had a target time to try and beat. He was a wee bit isolated during this period, but he also continued training and attending Taekwondo classes. He was something of an instructor, too. There were three main instructors there and from time to time Shane would be invited to run a session.

This was a paid job. Whilst being a Physicist at college and a student he would train alongside Tim and his sister, and go to the gym every day. Between August and October his question was about maintenance more than anything else. He was intending to pick up some more speed along the way. He would swim once a week to take the pressure off his joints, knees and ankles. Also, three mornings a week he would practice yoga and deep breathing.

As the time approached, his stress levels and sense of isolation increased. Being the autumn time of year and all, Shane got the moody blues. He began to get particularly aggressive as he realised that he was on his own for this goal. Nobody was in for it with him. Tim had gone off to training camp with the squad, and Suzanna was not interested to run another full-distance marathon. Shane was the lone crusader here. How he knew it.

It came to the time of departure and Shane caught the bus to Teeside airport at 7 o'clock one October morning. He had intentionally arranged to pick up his tickets at the airport and pay for them at the reception desk. The bus journey took one and a half hours to get there, so he was there by 8.30am, and the flight was due to leave at 11am. Already there were throngs of customers milling around the airport awaiting their turn at the luggage desk, or to collect tickets, etc.

Shane took his turn at the ticket desk. No problems. The queue died down a little and he got to the front.

"Hello, I am here to pay for and collect my return ticket to Amsterdam please. My name is Shane Jeffries and reference number is 23APSYZWJ83L."

"Mr Jeffries…yes, we have you here on our files. How would you like to pay please?"

"Would Mastercard be alright?"

She nodded and accepted the card from him. Within only one moment she replied:

"I'm sorry sir, but it appears that your card is frozen. Do you have any other means of payment?"

"How do you mean? Why would my card be frozen? I have enough credit left on it for my ticket."

Shane was beginning to get upset at this point, and his mood was darkening once again.

"Sir, if you have a problem you could always talk it through with security."

"Fuck security! Give me my ticket, you sordid cow!"

With that she pushed a button underneath the counter and within moments a team of four police officers were on the scene. At first it was just talk:

"Is there a problem, sir?"

Shane began to shout at them in Korean. He launched himself at one of the young officers and cracked him square in the jaw. Before he knew what was what he had been tackled to the ground and handcuffed with hands behind his back. All the while he was yelling obscenities at them. They held him there for several minutes until the dust had settled and then picked him up and frog-marched him to the security outpost round the corner with his baggage, too.

This was searched and Shane was informed that he was being arrested and detained for assaulting an officer and posing a terrorist threat at an International airport. He was suddenly in a whole world of trouble that he had not expected. He was thoroughly interrogated as to his why's and wherefore's at the airport in the first place. Although physically intact still, his ego and esteem had taken a severe battering from the experience. They discovered his emergency contact number and phoned it. It was his Suzanna.

On being phoned by the police, she realised that something had obviously gone horribly wrong. She would have come to bail him out almost immediately, but was told that it would take some time to clear him, as GBH was a heinous action to take. Shane was taken into custody at Darlington Police Station for one night. The next day, as the case became clear, Suzanna brought the last few day's mail with her for Shane to open. One was a letter from the bank.

'Dear Mr Jeffries,

We are writing to inform you that as of September 30th we have frozen your Mastercard account as a bill has been left unpaid for over five months now. As soon as the previous bill gets paid in full, your account will reopen and be ready to use once again. If you have any further questions please feel free to contact us on the above given phone number.

Yours Sincerely,

Bank Manager'

Shane could have screamed, or at least ripped up the letter. He looked at his sister "They could have told me before I got to the airport!"

She replied, "Don't worry, they told me all about it. Sorry about your marathon, that will have to wait until next year now. I guess you've landed in a quandary then, huh?"

They sat in silence for quite some time, mulling things over. Shane knew his dad would not be best impressed with his performance here at the airport, but he figured that it was necessary to face the music anyway.

And face the music he did. During his time in police custody they offered no consolation whatsoever, just leaving him with the sense of a faded victory. Up until that point, Shane had viewed his running the Amsterdam marathon as a metaphor for his prowess, his absolute vigour, and very essence of being an athlete. He was in good form, it had to be said. Although now he would sit in a stupor to recalculate and evaluate where he was at.

Suzanna laughed about it for the next week, which made matters worse, unkindly so; it had become a farce. Shane was not to so much as cross the start line at this event. The loss was his alone. He had been going alone since August, and he received very little sympathy, if indeed any at all. He wasn't after sympathy, he wanted results. These would come if only he had the go-ahead.

Having been blocked just like that this one time he resolved to dig deeper and become even more determined for the next year ahead. The two siblings would continue to compete in this way, as much for their own benefit as for the Team they were involved with; also for Tim, of course.

Suzanna had managed to spend time with their father and calmed him down. He didn't like to think that his son had been brought down by the constabulary for that reason. Not for any reason ideally, but this minor infringement would soon blow over and be done with. Mr Jeffries snr was worried that 'history would repeat itself' and leave the family with a disgrace case to deal with. Suzanna consoled him, telling him that the miscalculated event wouldn't end their time with the North Yorkshire squad. This appeased his mind and ego, at least in the immediate term. Shane received a stern word or two from his father and was warned that he may have his allowance cut were there to be any further shenanigans like that. Shane did not need to hear this twice.

So, on reflection, the year had been an achievement. They had run two major events in London and achieved well locally in the summer time. It would go without saying that had Shane been teamed up with a coach in October, the bank details would have been checked in due time and this whole brouhaha would probably not have occurred. He would not have been foolish enough to assault the officers, because he would have had company to keep him on the straight and narrow. At least that is how it seems in this marvellous thing called retrospect.

In effect, Shane had received the Royal Pardon from family, colleagues and club in next to no time at all and had been encouraged to keep on track and look ahead to the Half marathons in February 2012 with the club runners. He would soon have forgotten all about the incident. Moving on, that was the name of the game.

It got to December 2011, and Christmas was in everyone's mind. The Jeffries' family would have a family get-together. Their grandparents, uncles and aunts would all come to spend time together. The rota seemed to go round. Some years they all came here, and other years they all went to another's place.

Shane and Suzanna kept each other's moods up throughout. They just kept training, even on Christmas Eve and Boxing Day, just taking one day off for Christmas Day itself. Weight gain would not be on their own agenda if at all possible.

Next event would be a New Year dash, a New Year splash, and an attempt at some New Year cash involving a strip down to the minimals and a splash around North Bay, Scarborough, at the beginning of January. Prizes would be awarded for the most zany dressing habits, and for the quickest swimmers from point 'a' to point 'b'.

Shane entered for the quickest swimmer and damn near came off with the prize, but some other person pipped him by default; in fact, had made a grab at his legs near the end line. Nearly drowned him, but the judges only saw that the winner had won so that was the way it went. Shane made a protest, but had to be content with second place anyhow.

Suzanna entered for the zany costume category, she dressed as 'Beetlegeist' with yellow and black stripy stockings. This caused a stir amongst all the fellow-participants, and had some people in stitches. She won £25 for her attempts and even swam 100m in the costume before getting out of the very cold water, and back onto the beach. They were serving drinking chocolate and coffee on the beach and provided thermal blankets to minimise the possibility of catching hypothermia. She loved the craziness of it all.

Back into regular training they determined to run the City of York half marathon, the 'Brass Monkey', later in the month of January. Tim, too, entered this race and the three came together for the first time in months. None would win, or even make the top 10, but they utilised the event as a stretching pointer for the next time they would 'run to win'. Validly speaking, Tim could have won these meets if he had put his mind to it, or at least get a decent time and high position. Shane would aim for fitter, stronger, faster, and Suzanna would still remain content with a pb.

After the run in York, the three drove home together. They began to talk to each other:

"Well run, guys, you've done yourselves proud today", said Suzanna.

"Thankyou Suze, you angel, you too, you've done good!" replied Tim.

"Yeah, thanks Suze, couldn't be doing this without you guys. We're still a team, right?" inquired Shane.

"Of course we are! One for all and all for one – just like the three musketeers!" she projected.

"Aoooouuuuuuuuuuuuuuuu!" howled Tim in approval.

They laughed and drove on. Shane was driving, and preferred to concentrate on the job at hand. He wasn't the most social animal of the three, but was more practically orientated. Hence the Physics, the experiments, the athletics, the Taekwondo, and the moods when it came time to express what he would naturally do without talking too much. Shane could do stuff. Suzanna, on the other hand, being a girl, liked to talk a lot. Yes, she could run, but when an opportunity presented itself to verbalise, you could bet your bottom dollar that she would seize it and relish the chance.

Tim was often pensive. He was often quiet, reflective and something of an enigma. He was never particularly disposed to gregarious social activity. This would be something for others to concern themselves with. Just leave him to his training and all would be well.

When he had learnt of Shane's adventure back in October he felt guilty actually. Probably because he was the one with a coach and management guiding him forwards. Tim had offered nil support for Shane's marathon attempt. Well, strictly speaking, it would be his second attempt at this full distance event. Tim discovered that whilst he had had a coach he had been performing a whole heap better than when he was just on his own, as Shane had been.

It was understood that there had been a rough patch. Both siblings, Shane and Suzanna, had always been competitive, right from an early age. It began with the family pool table and the table tennis. Grades in school were bounced off one another, and it came as no great surprise to immediate relatives that their enthusiasms continued and grew into their athletic endeavours. Tim had become an extremely valuable appendage to their own endeavours. They welcomed him like a brother, and trained with him like a made man.

They wanted his success just as much as their own. The stratosphere was cast already, there would be no treading where one did not belong. Tim clearly belonged in amongst a higher league of athlete, Suzanna belonged at the restaurant and running triathlons, and Shane belonged in the lab, or running with the North Yorkshire squad. They all had good prospects for a bright future, even with the qualms and niggles that were evident from time to time.

Endeavours coupled with antagonism and challenge. 'There is no such thing as a problem', thought Shane, 'only challenges which are there to be overcome'. He could shift his mentality like that. He generally carried a positive psychology with him. With a bare minimum of emotional baggage, he had few hang-ups. His intangible mood swings would come and go, all the while they would clear up and he would make headway for the next thing, the next goal, the next endeavour. He could step up where needed. If asked, he would surely be there.

He had proven this to Suzanna on several occasions, and would again. Shane had taken a personal disliking to Benjamin Williams and didn't like the fact that every time they met he seemed to be hitting on his sister. Shane was convinced that Ben was gay. Whether this was true or not is another matter, but anyway, he had convinced himself that Ben was an outsider and not fit for his sister, but Suzanna did not particularly mind this attention that she received. Although, clearly, she had a crush on Tim, she would make no real complaint about the matter.

Shane held it as a personal grudge. This would no doubt unfold as time went by. Let's hope so, eh.

Shane had nobody in particular in his sights. He was something of a loner, hence his reliance on his sister's company and Tim's partnership. He was in no hurry whatsoever to hook up with somebody. He was genuinely contented to be training and keeping fit all the time. Figuring that it would make an inspirational story at the very least, he was happy to live like this.

After all, he had Suzanna and Tim who had come to rely on him as a close associate. This was surely the most valuable offering that there could ever be? If not, then Shane would find solace in science. He was determined as always, and would anticipate any encouragements that he ever received. Whether from fellow Physicists, or from athletes, Shane was wrapped in his own game by now. He was very much his own man.

Suzanna would go to work in Collage pretty much every day, and train pretty much every day as well. Her timetable was equally full. Her relationship with her brother had proved typically familial. Always there for him, even when the timing was a bit out, or inconvenient in some way. She had proved her loyalty after all by coming for him at Teeside that night in October.

They were bonded mainly by the prospect of bigger and better things to come. A brighter future, full of adventure and wonderment. Tim getting onto Team GB boosted their morale enormously. He was really on the team and would therefore stand a chance of going to London in the summer and winning a medal. If only he had the vote of confidence from his own parents. They still found him to be deluded, as parents do.

Shane and Suzanna had seen the whole process and now their efforts had paid off. Tim had qualified after the London Triathlon back in August, thanks to these two siblings. Without them in particular, his training would have had only half the effect that it did. Their rivalry had paid off up until now. And there were no signs that this was going to change.

Not in the immediate future if this could be at all helped. Shane and Suzanna had been plugging on for years by now with the triathlon, and now the regular training was kicking in. They were a team and were winning. This is what they would have wanted to happen. Their competitive nature was at play. The year had been productive to say the least, and now was their chance to step it up once again and experience a whole new level. Life as they could only dare dream about.

Name: Tim Richardson 'The Athlete'
Age: 21
DOB: 24th March 1991
Star sign: Aries
Height: 5' 10''
Weight: 10 ½ stone (87kg)
Eye colour: Green
Hair colour: Brown
Current hair style: Medium in length, rebellious styles to suit
Character: Wildcard with bags of enthusiasm. Believes he will win Olympic Gold!
Special relationships: looks up to Ben as mentor figure
Best friend: Shane
Special interests: Skating, BMX biking, Triathlon, Heavy metal/rock/grunge music
Favourites: *Food* ~ Steak and chips with onion rings, peas and French mustard,
Drink ~ Sparkling water, Michelob Ultra
Movie star ~ Tom Cruise, Tom Hanks, Jack Black
Movie ~ Mission Impossible
Bands ~ U2, Muse, Kings of Leon
Artists ~ Bono, Craig David
Clothes ~ Asics/Reebok athletic wear.
Career: J Sainsbury's Store Assistant, Team GB cycling athlete/triathlon

Name: Claire Halls 'The singer-songwriter'
Age: 23
DOB: November 4th 1989
Star sign: Scorpio
Height: 5' 6''
Weight: 9 1/2 stone (60kg)
Eye colour: Hazel-Brown
Hair colour: Black
Current hair style: Long and straight
Character: Highly intelligent, multi-lingual, talented musician. Creative extraordinaire, and a depressed diabetic.
Special relationships: love match with Charlie, Alex's licence allows her to perform in Collage
Best friend: Charlie
Special interests: guitar playing, singing, French, Spanish, musician song-writing
Favourites: *Movie star* ~ Jennifer Aniston
Movie ~ Along came Polly
Food ~ Caesar Salad Continental European,
Drink ~ Michelob Ultra or Chardonnay,
Bands ~ Atomic Kitten/Girls Aloud/Sugababes/The Saturdays/Westlife
Artist(s) ~ Alison Moyet, Sade, Ronan Keating
Clothes ~ special-knit green woolly jumper for the winter and summer dresses when hot.
Career: Professional musician

Name: Charlie Morris 'The Entrepreneur'
Age: 25
DOB: July 10th 1987
Star sign: Cancer
Height: 6' 2''
Weight: 15 stone (a muscular 95kg)
Eye colour: Blue
Hair colour: Blonde
Current hair style: Short cut, smart, neat
Character: Kool Kat, rolls with the punches. Bipolar and has picked up an ASBO for aggressive tendencies.
Special relationships: Going out with Claire
Best friend: Claire
Special interests: owns a tropical fish store 'Fish4U!'
Favourites: *Food* ~ Shepherd's Pie with green peas
Drink ~ San Miguel, Lucozade Sport
Movie star ~ Ben Stiller, Owen Wilson, Vince Vaughen
Movie ~ Starsky and Hutch
Band(s) ~ Metallica, Aerosmith, Guns 'n' roses, The Who
Artist(s) ~ Axl Rose, Roger Daltry, Jimmy Page
Clothes ~ Blue Jeans, plain white t-shirt, sunglasses and leather jacket (when the weather permits).
Career: Entrepreneur

Name: Shane Jeffries 'The Brother'

Age: 24
DOB: 23rd August 1988
Star sign: Virgo
Height: 5' 8''
Weight: 11 ½ stone (73kg)
Eye colour: Hazel-brown
Hair colour: Chestnut brown
Current hair style: parted at the left side
Character: serious scientist, liable to succumb to destructive mood swings. Asthmatic.
Special relationships: brother of Suzanna, Tim's training partner (triathlon athletes)
Best friend: Tim
Special interests: Desires the Nobel prize one day, Triathlon, and Taekwondo
Favourites: *Movie stars* ~ Jeff Goldblum/Russell Crowe
Movies ~ The Fly/A Beautiful Mind
Bands ~ Coldplay, Texas, Massive Attack
Artist(s) ~ David Gray, Nelly Furtado
Food ~ Domino's Pizza
Drink ~ Irn Bru
Clothes ~ Smart shirt and tie in order to appear respectable.
Career: Taekwondo instructor

Name: Suzanna Jeffries 'Shane's sister'

Age: 22
DOB: 18th December 1990
Star sign: Sagittarius
Height: 5' 10''
Weight: 10 stone (84kg)
Eye colour: Hazel-brown
Hair colour: Mousy brown
Current hair style: Medium-long wavey
Character: fun-loving, easy-going, open minded girl with epilepsy.
Special relationships: Shane's sister, Tim's confidante
Best friend: Tim
Special interests: people
Favourites: *Movie star* ~ Brad Pitt, George Clooney
Movie ~ Ocean's 11/Ocean's 12
Food ~ Haute Cuisine
Drink ~ Chateau Neuf de Pape
Bands ~ Evanescence, The Zutons, Take That
Artist(s) ~ Michael Ball, Leona Lewis, Gary Barlow
Clothes ~ Nike sportswear
Career: Waitress/Barista

Name: Benjamin Williams   'The Professor'
Age: 30

DOB: 27th April 1982
Star sign: Taurus
Height: 6' 0''
Weight: 14 stone (88kg)
Eye colour: Green
Hair colour: Dark brown-black
Current hair style: conservatively short
Character: Mature, mentor figure. A touch of OCD
Special relationships: Tim's adviser, owns a Cocker Spaniel called Pépé
Best friend: Pépé
Special interests: PhD Ethics Professor
Favourites: *Movie star* ~ Laurence Olivier
Movie ~ Lawrence of Arabia
Drink ~ Blackcurrant Ribena
Food ~ vegetarian lasagne with minted boiled potatoes
Bands ~ Beethoven/Mahler/Wagner symphonies, Radiohead
Artist(s) ~ Bob Dylan, Mozart, Sibelius
Clothes ~ Suit with shirt and tie.
Career: Ethics Professor

Name: Alex Davies 'The Restauranteur'
Age: 32

DOB: 23rd July 1980
Star sign: Leo
Height: 6'1''
Weight: 15 stone   (96kg and big boned)
Eye colour: Green eyes
Hair colour: Black
Current hairstyle: respectable
Character: entrepreneur, Owns and Manages 'Collage' and 'The Flaming Squirrels'- Dyslexic.
Special relationships: Wife Melanie (28), daughter Fiona (5) and Charlie (fellow entrepreneur)
Best friend: Melanie
Special interests: making all customers feel welcomed.
– Restauranteur of *Collage*
- Chief Barista at The Flaming Squirrels
Favourites: *Movie star* ~ Angelina Jolie & Keanu Reeves,
Movie ~ Lara Croft: Tombraider & The Matrix
Bands ~ Stereophonics, Guns n Roses
Artist(s) ~ Damien Rice, Alexandra Burke, Robbie Williams
Food ~ breaded mushrooms with garlic dip starter followed by roasted breast of chicken with chipped potatoes seasoned with paprika, and fresh spinach. For dessert, a Neapolitan ice-cream with chocolate crisps and wafer biscuits, plus complementary sparkler.
Drink ~ full bodied red wines eg Merlot
Clothes ~ Professional chefs regalia
Career: Entrepreneur/Restauranteur

Chapter 6
Pépé 1

Having recently fallen out with Shane over his attempted liaisons with Suzanna, Ben found himself in a quandary. "What to do," Ben asked to himself, "now I have messed up with Shane and Suzanna?" He knew that Charlie was too wrapped up in Claire to give any form of honest appraisal of the situation. However, Ben received some inspiration – being an Ethics professor he made a conscious effort to come up with an ideal solution to any given predicament.

"What am I to do?" asked Ben. "I have no friends. Ah - either that means the life of Riley on my own, or I could make a whole new world of friends. How to do this?" "Dogs are man's best friend," screamed the answer to Ben. "If a dog is man's best friend and my best mate just fell out with me, surely I should be thinking in terms of getting myself a canine companion."

Related to friendship and dogs in particular, Ben had decided 'in the absence of a true friend, gain a dog. In the acquisition of a dog – man's best friend – your true friends would come thick and fast.'

Ben had fallen out with Shane owing to making moves on his sister, Suzanna. Both siblings subsequently spurned him forthwith and called him names like geek, nerd, being an 'anorak'. In consequence to this loss, Ben went off in search of a true best friend. As it unfolded he acquired a Cocker Spaniel whom he named Pépé. They became truly inseparable. Known as 'Team Pépé' Ben and his dog, with new found friends, all teamed together and made a famous stronghold of friendship, times and tribulations.

"A canine companion? Why of course – I shall call him Pépé." "What kind of dog fits the name Pépé? How about a Collie (perhaps too frisky); probably 'Charlie' for a Collie. Or a Dalmatian? Probably 'Cobi' for a daffy Dalmatian. I would surely spend my time counting the spots on the Dalmatian. So Pépé for a Spaniel, yes a Cocker Spaniel would be best. That way I can focus on what is truly important in my life."

"Were I to get a Spaniel, I would walk, wash, play, teach, and socialise without having to concern myself with counting spots all day long. So on balance, I think that I would prefer to own a spaniel – not, however, a droop-eared Springer, more the playful Cocker breed. So, 'Pépé' my Cocker Spaniel – theorem to be tried and tested," Ben thought to himself.

Ben had been busy weighing up the 'to buy a canine companion, or not to buy one' dilemma. To buy a dog now of all times would have made sense however. 'What value…how much is a dog actually worth?' 'If I were to pay £375 now for a puppy dog does this monetary price truly reflect the actual life of an animal being?' 'Should I spend £375 now on Pépé the Cocker Spaniel puppy, or should I guard my treasure for alternate purposes?' Ben quizzed himself with these questions.

"I think that I value my friendship higher than some coin, so my conclusion is to go ahead with the acquisition and buy a pet dog, pay the vet's bills, pay for food, drink and accessories, and of course hygiene equipment. Pépé would be worth far more than money alone," Ben concluded.

The main theory for Ben was: 'Dog is man's best friend especially when man is spurned by ex-best friend's sister.' Mr Ethics PhD professor consciously decided to try and test this theory, so he went out looking through the 'pets for sale' columns and contacted the abandoned dog agencies before landing on his Cocker Spaniel Pépé. His French connections from family childhood days meant that he felt comfortable with the name Pépé.

He had been thinking about it long and hard, and subsequently had come up with some other theories too. He had devised the following:-

Theorem two: does money maketh man? Or does true friendship count above all other? If true friendship counts above all else, then let Pépé be my shining light. Let there be canine companionship through and through.

Theorem three: the lucky mascot…friendship and happiness. Every team/event has a lucky mascot such as Micha Bear for the 1980

Moscow Olympic Games, or Cobi the dog at the Barcelona Summer Olympic Games 1992. Do we as human beings have the innate right to own a lucky mascot for our selves, for our lives?

A lucky mascot makes for a happier life!

Theorem Four: dining is a communal experience – I would rather eat in the company of my dog than eat alone for a lifetime.

Theorem Five: health and wellbeing. Better to be healthy than unhealthy – and how to stay well?.....get company!

A canine companion maintains wellbeing – emotionally, physically and socially.

With these five theories Benjy determined to decide whether or not to buy a dog indeed. And, of course, 'yassir' – Benjy was strongly in concurrence with having a canine companion.

To bear in mind though, were a few facts. Ben had previously suffered as a result of misguided theories. Hence he had recently upgraded his life unto being ten times more diligent and ethical in his demeanour (although to himself he multiplied this figure by much more!)

Ben's Theories all added up to five theories that determined whether life was worth acquiring a pet dog or nay. "A canine companion be for life young sir," he reminded himself, "and that equals responsibility, hard work, trips to the vet's and constant supervision. There is more to this than fun and games alone, my friend."

So there it was, decision made. Then crunch time. Ben went to the breeder's to buy a Spaniel puppy from a litter of six. "I can't believe these five puppies will never see their brother again," said Ben.

"Oh, don't worry yourself about that, young man, the dogs have full confidence in their master – and so do we – I'm sure that you will provide a safe, clean home for the Puppy dog. Say again, what will he be called?" inquired the breeder.

"Oh - Pépé!" answered Benjy.

"A splendid name for a Spaniel Puppy, I'll say. Feel free to bring him back for visits now, won't you? Remember as well, the vet's surgery is most important, Benjamin. The vet will help support you in raising the puppy now. So, bless your heart, young man," said the breeder's wife as Ben strolled along the garden path with newly-acquired Pépé.

No sooner was Ben on the street with Pépé in his arms than some friendly passers-by grinned and passed comment: "Ooooh, how cute, what a sweety. You've got yourself a bundle of cuddles there, sir!" one lady commented.

Pépé was the kind of Cocker Spaniel who you knew was your true friend. Just one playful yap and a slobber chops and you would know who your friend was. Never mind the Chihuahuas, the Lhaso Apsos, the Jack Russells, the Terriers or the Whippets…Pépé was Ben's dog, his loyal best friend. Never mind the Alsatians, the Dobermanns, the English Shepherds, the Akitas, or the Rottweillers; Pépé brought all that he ever needed – love, loyalty and friendship. The Cocker Spaniel who meant everything to everybody – that is, within the 'crew' – and going out was never quite the same ever again.

Benjamin had an awful lot of forethought about getting a dog in the first place. Not least of which were his careful ethical decisions a) time, b) money, c) socialising, d) hygiene, e) vet health, f) sterilising (could I actually bear to do that?...really?), g) whatever else it is that dog owners need to consider before buying their first doggo. As it transpired, there was precious little else that could have brought more happiness to Ben in his dark days. Although a PhD, Ben found plenty of solitude in his ways and getting a canine companion proved just perfect for his wellbeing. With a little persuasion, who knows, maybe Alex would make exception in Collage for pet allowance?

As he lived in Scarborough, Ben's favourite occupation included the early morning starts taking Pépé for a walk on the beach before the rest of the world managed to stir their stumps. Every morning Benjamin would walk Pépé at 7am before breakfast, then a long walk at 12 noon before lunch and an evening walk at dusk for dog's duty.

Either that or a diversion into the park by the lakeside. Either way, the key for Ben was the early morning where the sun shone and exercise occurred just before breakfast time so that the day got off to a blissful start. Whenever Ben got back home there would be a welcome reception of jumps, barks, circles, toing-and-froing, and wholesome doggo behaviour.

Other favourite jaunts for walking Pépé would include the Cleveland Way clifftop footpaths by the coast, and the local Dalby forest pathways. Pépé particularly enjoyed playing ball games. Throw a Frisbee and doggo would go hell for leather to return it. Truly a healthy species.

When not wondering about more philosophical issues, Ben would contemplate a few things, one being his good friend Tim, remarkably, divided yet not torn between his acceptance onto Team GB and his trusted mentor Benjamin. Being older, wiser and fully qualified, Ben carried the wisdom of ages with him. A form of authority in conversation.

Tim could only regard this maturity as an aspiration for later in his life. Ben matured early where some folk never gave up going out drinking and wilding it up. Ben had the capacity to settle down to read books and journals then to analyse them, take them to pieces, mentally rip them to shreds, then to make a thoroughly considered resumé of the material just read. This feat had been known to impress numerous people, not least Tim.

Being a J Sainsbury's Management Assistant in his working hours, Tim would often come across Company documents and read through them. Being an intellect and close colleague, Ben agreed once in a while to go through them with him together and see how Sainsbury could improve. He even once wrote a memo entitled '101 ways in which to improve J Sainsbury's.'

Tim and Ben collaborated on two projects – J Sainsbury and Team GB/London 2012. Any literature that Tim needed further clarification with, he would just take along to Ben and then go at it with fine wires. "No need to knock," he joked.

Charlie was convinced that their mentor relationship was largely down to Tim going to visit Pépé. There was no objection to this in the group. In fact, on the contrary, everyone loved the fact that Ben went out with a definite non-academic decision to buy a pet dog. Suzy commented that his life would improve for it.

So Ben and Pépé, the in-team; only Alex needed further persuasion that the dog was a good idea. Alex being a busy man, father, husband and business-owner was no push-over when it came to persuasion. Ben concerned himself that there might be a new 'Pépé pie' on the menu if he tried too hard to push his luck or his chances. No, Alex loved the dog truly as well, but his firm policy was 'no animals in my restaurant'.

Ben knew in his heart of hearts that there would come a day when there would be *eight* friends sitting around the table in Collage. Until then "let there be no animosity amongst friends", he thought.

Charlie and Claire came to visit Ben one evening after work. "How do you train your Pépé dog?" asked Claire. Ben told her that he had been attending dog obedience classes and a few tricks were included with this. 'Sit', 'Lie down', 'roll over', 'Fetch', 'Heel' and of course a response to his name 'Pépé'.

Truly, the puppy dog altered the group dynamics somewhat. Before Pépé, Ben was a much more lonely character. Although a valuable friend and mentor to Tim already, it has to be said that Pépé affected the entire perception of him as a person. The perspective of a lonely bachelor suddenly became one of a real human being striving towards fulfilling friendship and meaningful relationships.

Suzy felt personally responsible for the fact that Ben went out to get a dog. "I spurned him," she repeatedly thought to herself. "Shane hates him now for making moves on me.....it's not his fault, after all what is more natural than a friendship trying to go one step further?...and then not. I must speak with Shane as a responsible sister and straighten him up. Poor Ben just can't go on with Shane acting up like this".

She determined to make up with Ben and get her brother back on good terms with him. Although Ben was serious about going out together, he felt somewhat rebuffed. He would take some time to come back round again, she just knew.

After all, had she accepted Ben's forward moves then they would actually be going out together, and maybe, just maybe, Shane would be more accepting of the fact, instead of all this nonsense about rejection, you know, the kind that causes consternation and pain. Ben, prior to this girl, had had only two girlfriends. Maybe it was this thought that turned Suzy off dating him…wanting somebody with a little more experience; or at least who acted as though he meant it.

Whatever it was that divided her emotionally from dating Ben, Shane felt pissed. Really pissed, as in rip it up and shit down your neck pissed. Nothing he did could either affect or change this in the immediate term or the foreseeable future.

Anyway, how did Shane fit in with Pépé? He didn't really. Maybe, only out of current emotional envy or hostility.

So Ben was rejected by Suzanna. To be honest, she found him too dull, too plain; too much of a geek or a nerd. This didn't meet her club requirements for a boyfriend. Ben knew that he would eventually stand a chance if he didn't give up hope. "Keep supporting the triathlons. Offer Tim a constant mentor. Try and get around Shane's animosity."

Although it hurt, having been single for seven years now, he knew not to give up trying. There would be somebody for him somewhere along the line. Ben was an eccentric through and through. Probably from spending so much time on his own rather than engaging in a social furore. His intelligence could not be denied, his lecturing skills admired by his students. But girls, as yet, didn't seem to care, not a jot, not an iota, not a wink or a nudge, not even a bat of an eyelids at that.

Ben knew too much for his own good. It all came pouring out in class. Put quite simply, his lack of companionship made him lonely so on his quest for company he figured that he couldn't go far wrong with a dog at home to talk to on an evening. Pépé knew this as well. He just knew his master's solidarity at home. So with this in mind the two of them got on like a house on fire, very well indeed.

Pépé was no pooper. Of course, he pooped. On a regular basis, in fact. But he was no party pooper. This Cocker Spaniel was rather a goer in the world. Every walk would be a true adventure, every smell, every sound, every movement seen, a whole panoply of discovery was to unfold before him; especially the walks on the beach. All the other dogs wanted to play together or to swim in the sea, or to fetch items from across the sand. This Cocker Spaniel would roll with glee on being granted an outdoor walk every morning and afternoon.

Fortunately, Ben owned a cheap Vauxhall Astra so transportation between places was feasible as well. Although he didn't know it, Ben was convinced that one day soon he would win the National Lottery so he played twice a week. The most he'd ever won in a week was £10 but he never gave up hope. He had in fact written a *Masterplan*, a *Blueprint*, what exactly to do with the winnings once they came in. One plan directly involved Pépé. 'Get a new friend.' Well, he hadn't won the lottery jackpot quite yet, but he had won a canine companion.

Winning the lottery would change the world for Ben. For a start, he would move house and buy a decent car, a brand new BMW, or Lexus as an option, so long as the fuel efficiency met global requirements and caused minimal pollution in the atmosphere. So long as his dog could sit or lie down comfortably, and so long as the passenger seat spelled out 'here shall sit your sexy lady, so do not fret ever again' he would be content with that.

Ben and Pépé were both well known in the neighbourhood. He had some who doubted him as well, however; some who deemed him a social freak, a goon, a weirdo, a crazy camper, or some such notion. He never displayed any signs of aggression although he felt a bit torn when comments would come from time to time.

Actually, time had changed things. Pépé broke the ice for him and Suzanna one day when they met by chance at a cafe. When they met that morning she squealed with delight…

"Whatchya got here then Mr?"

"His name is Pépé."

"Isn't he sweet, isn't he gorgeous?"

"My best friend. *Only* friend in fact," having a dig at Suzanna.

"Well, that's really something. Mr Ben's got himself a spaniel. What kind of spaniel Benjy?"

"A Cocker Spaniel."

"Why, I bet he was expensive. How much did you pay for him?"

"I shouldn't say really, but I will. Pépé cost me £350 as a puppy dog. Five months from new born."

"I say. You got yourself a deal there, Mr."

Suzanna continued "Can I get you anything to drink? I was just going to have a coffee for fifteen minutes."

"OK, that would be lovely, thanks. A coffee, too, please. Thanks", Ben replied.

Ben's hopes were picking up by now and he figured that Alex must be working at Collage today as some new barista served them both coffee at their table in the cafeteria.

Ben and Suzanna sat together with Pépé at their feet for an hour, idly chatting. This led Ben to believe that the previous spurning was to do with her brother's animosity towards him. Shane was in fact jealous. Ben already had a career which had begun to take place. Shane's dream of a Nobel prize meant that anybody with intelligence either represented a blessing and source of instruction to him, or a threat and a cause for cynical resentment. In this case he hated Ben's guts for possessing intelligence. Shane knew that ethically, Ben could teach him anything at all, but that fact was not enough.

Perhaps, there could be a new breakthrough here? But no, the triathlon kept the two siblings together, and Shane was jealous that Tim approached Ben for mentoring. Shane was outclassed by Tim and by Ben and he resented that fact. All the more because he trained so damned hard.

Tim was a Superstar as far as the County were concerned. He had twice finished the Great North Run in the top twenty. Running a half marathon in 1hour 15minutes was in his field of competence. Shane was more a 1hour 25 minute man at his best.
What a peach for an athletic rivalry!

Anyway, back to the dog. There was now a case file of proof and evidence that Pépé had restored full confidence in Benjamin as a friend.....

1) passers-by made friendly gestures towards the pair of them on a regular basis.
2) Ben received visitors especially on account of the Cocker Spaniel companion.
3) Being an ethics lecturer, Ben brought canine ethics into his college classes.
4) Suzanna had made up to Ben as a worthwhile friend
5) Charlie and Claire made special efforts to be with Ben often.

Evidence to the contrary......
1) Alex's restaurant 'Collage' was strictly 'no pets' and certainly 'no dogs allowed inside'. Collage happened to be the chief focal and meeting point for the group of friends.
2) Shane remained hostile and cynical towards Benjamin out of fraternal protective interests towards Suzanna.
3) Pépé's poop caused a constant responsibility.

So, already the two were on better terms by now because of the dog. They had met at the café and had begun to strike up an intrinsic rapport like never before. That chance encounter could change everything for Ben. Would he now stand a chance? Would the troubles ease off? Could it continue in this light now it had started a new way?

Pépé just hustled and bustled about the place, being a lively puppy dog, not really caring for a 'who's who?' or a 'what may I do Sir?' He behaved in entirely puppy dog fashion. That's why everyone loved him. And wherever the dog was, so was Ben.

A fair play scheme. Pépé had quite literally saved his day. No more lonely, morose hours pondering in the darkness. He now had company, and that was permanent. One man and his dog.

Ben had seen the show on telly from time to time about the sheepdog trials and seemed intrigued by the level of intelligence that both Collie and farmer demonstrated during the whistling – go thither, come hither show.

Ben was officially a happy chappy. A whole world happier than six months previously, anyhow. "Tantaraa, tantaraa," sounded the trumpets as Ben walked with an air of pride around the campus. At least that is how he imagined it at the time.

The time was now and there was no time to lose. Not now, not then, not ever again. No time for procrastination. Not in Ben's book. He had a fertile imagination. "God bless America! Vive la France! Viva España! God save the Queen!" Ben thought to himself feeling positive within.

He had his ups and downs still, but on the whole he was very pleasantly optimistic. This rubbed off on his students during class. Some days people would come to see him in his office and congratulate him on his delivery and content. Some students requested advice and direction – most in fact – whilst the occasional few would come to see him with a 'groundbreaking' theory about how to change the face of the world.

The former type were welcome guests in their droves whilst the latter would generally be reprimanded and told to reevaluate their theories as they were some 'crackpot' scheme or other. Some big ideas came through from time to time and Ben had the critical job of managing these students to their practical application. This was no mean feat, by any standards.

At least he would know what to say regarding his ethics and subject matter. Ben had a key role to play here. He had many students and regarded Tim as being amongst his own. Even though he looked upon Tim as being in a different league of sorts, he stood by the viewpoint that he was a student figure doing his thing in the world.

"Hey-ey-ey-ey-ey-ey-ey," Ben mumbled to himself upon reading one student's thesis. He knew that he had come across a rare piece of quality. The introduction presented the case, and the development saw it explored from every angle, and the conclusion thoroughly impressed him. Ben sat back and lit his pipe. This he enjoyed from time to time; moments of philosophic deliberation and contemplation often accompanied his pipe-smoking moments. He felt to be very much Master of Ceremonies in these moments; a dignified gentleman leading a noble existence in his universe.

Times were moving on and things had changed progressively a little over the days as they passed, some things for the better, some for the worse. One day, Tim came to see Ben and they started a conversation:

"Wow, what an awesome trip I've just had, man!"
"How do you mean?"
"Well, dude, I was just jogging down the street training when I passed a crowd of gorgeous chicks."
"Oh, is that it?"
"No, man, it gets better.....they began to chant like they were cheerleaders or something - singing and dancing and jumping around....."
"...I was chased for half a mile by two of them along the street."
"Wow, you must be nervous then?"
"No way, what a trip! That's the first time that's ever happened to me!"
"Hmmmmm, so what a day", uttered Ben.

They grinned about the matter like little oiks for a moment, and then Ben carried on:

"Is that all you came for? To boast about that? Or, what can I do for you Mr Richardson?" he asked.

"Oh, de nada, señor. Just to let you know that, and an update on the training front. You know what? I think Suzanna likes you Ben. Yes, in truth, it's just that thing with Shane, isn't it? You know, I can see it properly. When did you last meet?"

"Oh, actually we met recently at the café, with Pépé, too. We had a good chat and left on a good note."

"See, what did I tell you?" said Tim to Ben.

"Well, I don't want any trouble, mind," Ben replied.

"No need to be such a wet dweeb, Benbo! She likes you and you stand a chance. I know these things…we train together."

"Ohhh, ok, we'll see what comes of it then".

"Yeah. Just let a good thing slip away from your fingers? Nooooo man! You've got to get in there and seize your opportunity while you have the chance."

Ben stood there in rapt consternation for a moment. He squeezed his chin and his eyes became that of a predator, like a lion. He was making the transition from humble failure to man of distinction with credentials attached.

He looked back towards Tim, and they started talking once again:

"You're right - dammit man! I knew it. Goodness gracious, it seems so apparent now you say the words. I must make the most of it and seize the day – Carpe Diem as they say."

Tim nodded in approval at his mentor's revelation. They had a moment of understanding between them, and then Tim made a conclusive statement with:

"Well, glad to be of service, Sir. Must dash, I have to be at Sainsbury's for the evening shift."

They parted company and Ben remained pottering around at home. Oh, one more word for Tim whilst visiting was that the dog received a pat to the head and an instruction to 'sit!' from him. Pépé obediently obeyed this command and was rewarded with a few biscuits to chew on.

Ben was really delighted to hear from Tim himself that he stood a chance with Suzanna. This added to his cheery self. He felt to be a hit with the ladies all of a sudden, a real ladykiller, a man who was desired by all. He thought 'Boy, oh boy, I'm really a fighting man now,' as he had got quite fired up over the idea. He was ready to go out and conquer the world. 'Ben's my name and my life is my game' he uttered gleefully.

He meant business and was most serious about the matter. Tim had established within him a certain optimism for an inevitable event rather than an inkling of a faux pas. Their conversation had been a turning point in his thinking. And now would come the time to make the next move.

As it happened, a few days passed and Tim had arranged a training date with Suzanna at the swimming pool one morning. He decided to get the ball rolling for Ben, and said a few words to her:

"You know Suzanna, I wouldn't be where I am now were it not for Ben. He has really made a big difference to my training fitness and psychology."

"Yes, he's alright, isn't he. I love the puppy - really cute, mind. When will you see him again?" she asked Tim.

"More to the point, Suze, when will *you* see him again? You know I think there could be something good going on there!"

"Welllll, you shouldn't embarass me like that Tim. What will be will be and we can only see what comes of it. Especially with my darned brother. He's a real spanner in the works, you know."

"I could always speak to Shane next time we meet. I reckon I know exactly what to say to him," Tim replied.

"Oh, I'm not so sure about that, Tim. He's a sticky customer at the best of times. I should know. He's been my brother for over twenty years now."

They got on with their training, and swam for one and a half hours. Suzanna knew that she would meet Ben again sometime soon and hoped they would be able to get along just fine once again. Tim was puffed out and exhausted from the session so went to change and go home again.

It was she who made the move. She had got Ben's phone number from Tim, and later that afternoon made a surprise call:

"Hello Ben, it's me Suzanna."
"Oh, my. What a surprise. Well, how do you do?"
"I'm very well thankyou. I just called to see if you'd like to go out sometime for a walk or something?"
"Oh, well, that would be great. I could bring Pépé along if you don't mind."
"No, silly. That would be terrific. I am a fond admirer of your dog."

"Ok then, so let's meet at the park tomorrow afternoon at 1.30pm and we shall take a stroll for an hour, if that's alright."

"Yes of course. That would be simply terrific. So, until tomorrow then – hasta mañana!"

"Yes indeed – ciao ciao," Ben concluded before hanging up.

This breakthrough delighted him further as his hopes were coming to life. His dog was doing the trick. New friendships, new times, as good as gold. He hardly slept a wink that night. The next morning flew by. Breakfast was a botched job, he burnt the toast in fact, and spilt his coffee down his shirt, to which he responded with an anguished groan "Doh!" in the style of Homer Simpson.

Then at a quarter past one in the afternoon he put the collar on to Pépé and the two of them set off to the park. There she was, at half past one on the dot, ready and waiting, wearing a bright and colourful shirt and open jacket for a sunny day.

"Hello," understated Ben, typically British in style.

He gave her a kiss on both cheeks (more continental all of a sudden) and the two began their afternoon stroll together.

"What a fine day it is today," mentioned Suzanna.

"Yes, indeed, hardly a cloud in the sky," Ben replied.

They smiled at the prospect of something new happening now. But what was to actually unfold? Who could tell? Who would know? Could anybody predict the future, after all?

"You're looking in great shape, Suzy"
"Thankyou. You're not too bad yourself"
"Yeah, I like that, as though I train every day, like you," Ben said almost with a hint of sarcasm.
"Well, I gotta keep fit, you know"
"Fitness is as fitness does," he went on. "They say that true fitness is in the recovery period".
"That's interesting. Yeah, I have heard that before"
"So you train in the morning and then come out walking in the afternoon – that makes you one fit cookie in my book," Ben complimented her.
"You're not wrong, Mr Ben – gotta keep on top of these things now, you know," she giggled.

They walked in the sunshine in Peasholm park and round by the seashore promenade for the afternoon stroll. Pépé was on his best behaviour and caused some intrigued glances as they walked. Ben had resolved inwardly to keep at it, to keep the side at work, to keep up the British spirit. Life was beginning to look up once again, especially more so that his relationships had begun to take a significant path after all those years of solitude, loneliness, and abject misery.

He had a job, he had a dog, and now he was on the verge of having a girl. Things were definitely looking up for him, in truth. 'Life could have been worse, so much worse,' he knew. He was lucky, one of a privileged few. He was beginning to feel complete, a whole man, a real person.

Yes indeed, in these times for Benjamin Williams and his dog Pépé, things were working out just fine. Team Pépé a-go-go, 'you'd better look out, you'd better watch out, cause they're gonna getcha; One man and his dog,' 'ahhhh' smoking a pipe, the master of sophistication.

Chapter 7
Battle of the Bands

There was soon to be a battle of the bands competition in Vivaz bar. There were to be eight different bands playing in alternate styles of music, from the more easy-listening folk-rock of Seachimp, through blues to metal and punk-rock. One band in the battle, called Locust Hotel, played some heavier music jam-packed full of angst and social commentary.

Claire was already a regular performer at Collage by now. Some of these bands had whole tours behind them, under their belts. Locust Hotel for example, had played the entire local circuit by this time and had toured Northern England as well including the Cavern in Liverpool.

Their experience put Claire on edge somewhat. She was entirely a local lass. Would they be the winners who would scoop the recording contract? But maybe the winners would be those with wider experience. Maybe she would be a bag of nerves by the time Seachimp got to play. All these possibilities. She knew that she simply desired to win the recording contract and a cheque for £1000.

Some of the bands were rock orientated, some soul/gospel, some jazz, some blues, so a wide range of music was there to be performed by the artists at the Vivaz bar that evening.

She hated trash heavy-metal and held a worst nightmare fear that a band like this would win the contract and not Seachimp.

Life was full of bastards. Claire knew that already from her time in hospital. Since she had met Charlie her world had started to come together properly as though the pieces of a jigsaw puzzle were beginning to come together to form the whole beautiful picture.

The fact that Seachimp were invited to play at all at the battle of the bands renewed her self-confidence in herself and also in the band's material. Seachimp were being given some airtime beyond their usual spot at Collage. Plus with the chance to win a potential record contract she felt like good stock.

Charlie already knew Simon, the lead-singer of Locust Hotel, from various Scarborough haunts. They would go out for drinks together and discuss business propositions and means to proceed. How best to tackle an album? A new track? A new venture?

So Charlie knew Simon from the Scarborough circuit and Claire was dating Charlie. Hot competition for a winning spot at Vivaz bar was approaching. Would this jeopardise the way things were already? Who would come out on top? Would there be any love lost as a consequence? If so, could it be healed over?

Enough of the hypotheses for now, on with the show; dog eat dog. Simon sacked his bass player for complacency. That's what you get when the original crew were lined up and made a go of things and one person gets out of line too often. In this way things fell by the wayside. There was no room for this to be happening at all. So there we had it – a dog eat dog world.

The build-up to the battle of the bands. Behind the scenes Claire and Charlie were snogging furiously and intermittently. In between times the other bands were playing to the crowd. The event was being recorded for posterity. A local film crew were in the bar making a film of the event. Sound and Vision classed as A-important here in Vivaz.

The judges were to decide based on four leading categories: and in no particular order they were: 1) audience response, 2) originality of material, 3) quality of sound, 4) ability to communicate. Each band got to perform five songs prior to judgement.

In this way, there was a maximum ten points per judge allocated per song. So a total maximum of thirty points for each of the three songs, four categories, three judges. Thus the rules were formulated in this way.

First up:- a soul jazz set-up to start the show. A lead female singer on top of keyboard, acoustic guitar and percussion. She sang with spirit, with heart. There was enough emotion there to get the music to cut to your very core. In total she received 22 points from the judges' panel.

Next, second-up:- some pop-rock. Lead and rhythm guitars, bass guitar, vocalist on lead and drums. They surprised nobody. The 'Snappers' they had called themselves. The judges went by audience reaction and subjected them to a cruel 16. Due to over-familiarisation with the style one would believe.

Third-up:- a heavy-metal rock band. A spin-off from Aerosmith, Led Zeppelin, the Little Angels, or Metallica. They had written their own material. A very rousing performance (or deafening depending on how you look at it). Their credentials ran high, with a touring history behind them as well. Judges awarded 24 points onto this band.

Fourth-up:- none other than Seachimp. Claire had, by now, finished snogging Charlie and the band arrived on the stage. No nerves – cool as cucumbers. Being an original folk-rock setup, the judges took all criteria on board. There was great favour here. Seachimp were granted 28 points.

Fifth-up:- an unknown acoustic duo playing covers. Rock, soul, pop, blues. Unoriginal but technically demanding. The judges granted a score of 21 points in total. The bands were being held on tenterhooks by the judges' secret scoring system.

Sixth-up:- a visiting Norwegian band. They had electric fiddle, harmonica and big bass, doing Bluesy material and folk too. Fun stuff for all, but not a high scorer. They were granted 20 points in total.

The big number seven:- Locust Hotel. As an entertainer and first-rate performer, Simon sang from the depths of his soul. They raised the roof, raised their game, adrenalin pumping through all present. Judges took a shine and gave them 28 points, a first-place tie for which a one-song sing-off would be necessary.

Last but not least, number eight:- that night at Bar Zero, a standard rock set-up had deigned to enter the competition. Electric guitars, drums, bass, and screaming harpie as vocalist. No big score though.

They got harpooned and cut to pieces by the judges. Just 12 points. They were not good.

All this was captured by the film crew as well. And now the judges announcement. The scores were added up and thrown together. Then:

"We have a tie! A first-place between Seachimp and Locust Hotel, each with 28 points - we will have to be having a final one-song sing-off .... one final song each and we will decide the winner from this."

Rob, the bass player in Locust Hotel declared "Fuckin' ape-shit man, we should have won already!" He felt nauseously complacent.

Two completely contrasting styles of music in show. Punk rock versus Folk rock in the final show-down for a recording contract, £1000 cheque and a notoriety unparalleled in Scarborough. Who would come out on top?

Charlie suggested to Claire "sing that song that you sang me that time 'Walkin' The Line,' That'll get you the contract – guaranteed."

"Yup, that's the one I had in mind." The band formed and kicked into the song with gusto. It knocked off every man and woman's cleanest cotton socks. Everyone went wild with enthusiasm for Seachimp.

Then came the anticipation for the next song. Locust Hotel took to the stage and they broke into a punky rendition proclaiming youthful angst and melodrama. This song also grabbed the world's attention. Simon gyrated and the crowd grinned as the song progressed.

Only, the bass player then proceeded to trash his guitar on the stage. He flung it into the amps, snapping the D string. Just flipped completely. Thinking it would give them more sex appeal, he rocked out.

The crowd rocked too with mirth, shock, approval, disapproval, laughter, gasping, and disbelieving. They were a mixed bunch. Then, after a communal moment, came the judges' decision.

"There is no easy choice when it comes to declaring the champions. Both performances proved exquisite, exciting, passionate, enthusing. We have come to the conclusion however, that this year's Battle of the Bands champion is being awarded to the band with the originality, the crowd pleasers, the means and wherefores.......drum roll......we have decided to award the top prize and contract to......Seachimp! Congratulations one and all - a spectacle to behold and remember."

With that, the band went absolutely crazy, mental, hideously euphoric. They were delighted. Claire returned to Charlie yelling, "we did it, we really did it!" and they embraced like two grappling bears together.

Seachimp had actually won the recording contract and the cheque for £1000. This would mean that Claire could move onwards from Collage alone. On to greater things. They could now produce an album, a CD. Fantastico! Seachimp were up for higher bounty now.

Locust Hotel were fuming. Simon had a go at Rob "Why the chuff did you do that Rob? You complete and utter nobhead! What were you thinking?"

If it hadn't been for that show of instrumental disrespect Locust Hotel could have won the contract. They all knew that. "That's it, Rob the nob, you're fired - You're out of it, you're sacked - It's over!" yelled Simon.

"What for? I was doing the band a service" he petitioned.
"For complacency" shouted Simon.
"Bastard!"

Rob realised that Simon had meant it as band leader. The band now required a replacement bass player. Dog eat dog – Simon had sacked Rob from the very spot he had helped create.

Back in Claire's camp there were celebrations. "We made it, we really made it - Champions of the world!"

Charlie hung around the bar whilst the bands packed up their stuff, then Claire and he walked home feeling excited and turned on by the fact of what had just occurred.

"Think of what this actually means now. I can make a new album and sell it in HMV for £12.99. There is media coverage of the event. We're heading for the big time, baby!"

As they entered the house they embraced and made their way up to the bedroom. There they relaxed and began to get it on together. At first they kicked off their training shoes and then began slowly, but gradually, as emotion overcame them, to get truly passionate.

Claire had been wearing denim skirt with delicate coloured blouse and a green-grey cardigan on top to perform in. Claire began to peel off her clothing piece by piece. As the two lovers entwined their limbs together, Claire unzipped her denim skirt and Charlie took off his Levi jeans. He had been wearing jeans and a t-shirt underneath the sweater before they embarked on mission love-session.

Then she ripped off Charlie's sweatshirt jumper which she had bought him only recently when they left home to go out shopping together. Giorgio Rivera the brand, a sexy and fashionable orange-yellow top bought from the department store.

Claire allowed Charlie to relieve her of her own cardigan and t-shirt. The two rapidly became topless together embracing in the heat of the moment, admiring their slim and fit physiques. Claire's breasts proved young, nubile and slightly more than a handful for Charlie, whilst his abdominals and pectorals were a positive playground for her to admire. Charlie was a keen gym keep-fitter during the daylight hours.

Right down to their last remaining garment of underwear the pair of lovers lost all sense of inhibition and truly got passionate together.

As Charlie gently caressed her breasts, teasing Claire's nipples in between his middle finger and thumb, Claire began to get hot and moist between the thighs. Moaning with anguish and sumptuous anticipation of the love-making to come, Claire began to massage Charlie's ever increasing sausage with her left hand, just softly, but firm enough to cause an excitement and a stirring of the loins.

Her hair flowed silky soft, smooth against his spare hand and face as they began to pet, kissing each other on the lips, nose and nibbling the ears. Claire cupped her hand to the back of Charlie's head and pulled his mouth firmly onto hers and they progressed into a long deep French kiss, tongues probing curiously around each others mouth. Exploring her pearly white teeth and tasting her fresh, minty breath was never so appealing as now for Charlie.

The kiss lasted 12 minutes long although neither partner counted the time, their love-episode following a purely instinctual pattern, movements of their body intertwining throughout. As though the two were afloat on an astral beam of joy and ecstasy, they gradually eased themselves onto the soft, springy bed and embraced with continuous exploration as though the two had never before been this intimate, every session seeming to be a new adventure for them.

Claire's hair smelt of sweet summer meadows and her touch was as a gentle nymph of the forest. As her hands ran over Charlie's head and upper body, firmly pressing against his masculine pectoral muscles, gripping his manly bicep-tricep complex, she gained a thrill and profound sense of satisfaction from his erecting monument.

Both came prepared for the occasion so she unrolled a natural condom down the length of his cock and further teased him with her masturbatory gestures before they engaged in full intercourse together. He entered her body as a hot knife slides through ice-cream, sexual feelings running rife through the pair flying high on the plain of love together. Their session remained intimate, tender yet entirely meaningful between the two partners.

At the point of climax as she was driven to orgasm by him she was yelling out, 'Oh God, Oh God I'm there….Charlie you're the one, I love you, oh God this is so good!' They remained lying together in a hot, sweaty yet entirely contented state for a full 25 minutes afterwards before Claire went to take a shower and reemerged in her dressing gown to chat with the blessed-out Charlie.

"Always remember, we're a team," uttered Claire as they lay there."
"I know that, babe"
"I just wanted you to know that from my own lips….."
"…..you know, so you actually know it properly not just a conjecture."
"Claire you look so horny when you cum…"
"….I just wanted you to know that properly, you know….."
Claire hit Charlie with a pillow. "Silly."

Mellow conversation resumed between them as they discussed their plans for the next week. The day was Sunday and they had just begun to realise what a recording contract could actually mean for them both. They had just spent the entire night locked in each other's arms; and legs; and whatever else, too, come to that.

"The lyrics made good sense to me. Yeah, what was the line?.."
"..hmmmmm."
"Oh, that's it – life will never stay the same for this day or the next, so jump out and put aside all that had you vexed".
"I love that line, makes me laugh as well when I think about it, that is"
"Yeah, chick, whatever, I know; sounds a bit weird to me. I enjoyed the melody more than the lyrics though. Here's a word in French for you, hun. When I first saw you I thought to myself 'Mignon!'…"
"…know what it means?....'Cute'"
"Ooooh, that's such a word. I like that one".

The two went on for a while talking about their weekend social and what to do next week.

Claire now had a line-up of forthcoming gigs in local pubs/ restaurants and cafés, as well as an album to record with Seachimp. This prize was her first major coup in all her life, a major breakthrough. Alex, from *Collage*, still had an ongoing line-up of cabaret acts, poetry readings from time to time, and weekly gigs on a Saturday evening, where she would usually give a performance. The invite was open.

Claire and Charlie hit the group-news headlines with their relationship together. As it progressed they were able to embark on a youthful, liberated and liberating relationship throughout those cold winter months. They had come on so far since leaving the hospital over a year ago. The two got on famously.

They had been accepted as being together by now. Nobody was going to alter that fact. They had come together as a consequence of hard times and had really begun to stick together like superglue would bond card to paper. This was established and the crew were beginning to expect them to appear together whenever they went out.

Some weeks passed by and nothing out of the ordinary happened during this brief period. Then one day Claire suddenly had more than they both had bargained for. Claire had missed her period and had subsequently been to the doctor's for a check-up. The Doctor tested her and discovered that she was pregnant. This would change her life forever. Now with a recording contract on the one hand and a developing foetus on the other what would she ever do? Would they have a baby together? Would they have an abortion? It seemed so soon after all her hardships to be making that sort of decision and they came together in a serious way.

Alex talked to Charlie and figured that if they were really serious together then he had a business, Claire had a contract, they could have the baby and make a life work together. Charlie was OK with that idea. He was mature for his age and actually valued responsibility. He figured that an additional member to his life would be an essential component to fulfilment. He needed to speak to Claire. Was this too early for such an eventuality?

Claire was still very young. But not heartless. She would not feel too happy about the prospect of an abortion. In fact, she figured that even though the baby would have been an accident, so to speak, she may benefit from a fuller life and thus take her mind off her personal problems and onto a far greater external cause: motherhood, parenthood. They would need to get married. Oh, my God!

"Charlie, what are we going to do?" she plaintively asked.

"Be calm, babe – we have a decision to make. Do we have an infant now and make a new family together? We are both old enough for this and wise enough, and have decent lives to boot. Or do we back down from this life's greatest challenge?"

"I feel so stupid. We used protection as well. Why did this have to happen? I need time on my own to think this through."

With that Claire left the building and went for a walk in the park. She spent the next two days cogitating and thinking about having a baby. She decided that an addition to her own misery would cause a happy conclusion. After all, one need only walk around town on a typical afternoon to see all the other young ladies with their pushchairs and prams. She would be seen as normal and would fit in perfectly with the status quo. Maybe this would be just the ticket.

So she went back to Charlie and they sat down together and they talked.

"Charlie, I'm going to have your baby!" said Claire.
Charlie took a deep breath and feeling braver than ever before replied "Claire, I just want you to know that we are in this together - I'm with you all the way."

The pair sat together for an hour in silence, Claire with her head on his shoulder and Charlie rubbing her back. This would be the beginning of a whole new ball-game for them. They knew that they would have to go to the registry office soon and sort out all the details of a communion together.

It was while they were eating out at a local restaurant that Charlie decided to take affirmative action. During the course of the evening he suddenly popped down on one knee and asked Claire "Claire Halls – we're in this together. We've come a long way recently. I love you; will you marry me?" To which she replied "Charlie Morris, you never cease to surprise me. Yes, I will marry you!"

The proprietor brought out a bottle of champagne and the whole restaurant applauded the two fiancées. They felt like something real was occurring for the second time in such a short space of time.

At last, the life of Claire Halls was forming in to something beautiful. Just as surely as a pretty butterfly forms within the ugly caterpillar cocoon, her cocoon was now over and she was sprouting wings. Just as surely as a valuable pearl comes from the sand-irritated oyster, Claire Halls was producing the goods. She was now a recording artist with an entrepreneur man in her life, and a crew of close associates to keep her on track or at least to hear of her news as it arose.

Alex was the first to hear of their engagement together. He immediately felt jealous that they hadn't been in Collage during the proposal. Only briefly, however. He ordered Melanie to prepare some words of wisdom for them, or especially for Claire. She was very clever and knew exactly what to say to her. She gave an inspiring speech and told her to keep a track of her dreams, even with a little one on the way. This would not result in a tramp on the streets, everyone decided.

Charlie knew how to get extra finances already. He had some old, collectable magazines and antiques at home. He would sell them on ebay when the time came. There was bound to be a buyer, anyhow. Most things could be bought or sold on ebay at this time in our marketing history.

He was a business-man and would rely on his instincts to get as much financing as possible. What would they call the little one? This would be decided in time. Still early days for that kind of decision to be made.

Claire's pregnancy would change her world, though not in a bad way. This would be the second dramatic change in her life within a two month period of time. She had Charlie to support her, Melanie to engage with pearls of wisdom, and the rest of the crew to sympathise.

She had been going out with Charlie for 18 months by the time that he proposed. Not too long by anyone's standards, but long enough for them to realise that what they had should not be wasted into thin air.

This was a blessing and not particularly disguised at that. Everybody knew what was going on. So a competition, a recording contract, a night of passion, and now this. Claire was actually happy now, a happy bunny. She felt that her life was making sense at last. As though something important had been missing and now was found.

The facts were that since she and Charlie had met at Occupational Therapy, so much water had passed beneath the bridge. Charlie had made a pact not to talk about any of their previous trauma together, figuring that it would be preferable to focus on the new positive influences and events that the two had stumbled across.

In fact, funnily enough, Charlie had come across Simon once again from the band Locust Hotel. They got talking and Simon went on to express his warmest, sincerest and heartfelt congratulations. Upon learning of Claire's newfound status he didn't bat an eyelid, just asked what they would call it. "Too early," Charlie replied.

Simon said, "I've been looking for a keyboard player for the band."

"Oh?"

"Since we got rid of Rob on bass someone else stepped in. A couple of songs need a synthesizer or electric keyboard to jazz them up a bit".

"That would sound cool, man".

"Yeah, and not just that, but we've been offered some gigs around the UK…Glasgow, Liverpool, Birmingham, Leeds".

"Sounds like you're going for it!"

"Yes, sir – the band is up for a bit of groundbreaking touring. I hope that Glasgow's not as rough as reputed. I wouldn't want to provoke a riot in a bar".

"Haaa haaa haaa", Charlie laughed with pride at the prospect.

They got on superbly whenever they met, but didn't meet too often, actually. Simon came across as being hard, smart and good with words. Charlie came across more as an innovator. Especially with ideas for Fish4U! Simon told him that it sounded too much like a fish and chip shop for a Friday night takeaway, but what's in a name? Charlie didn't mind that comment anyway and carried on doing whatever he was doing. They chatted and went to the pub for a pint.

When they had finished their meeting, from a chance encounter in town, both continued on their separate ways. Charlie came home to Claire, Simon went home to walk his Border Collie.

The organisers of the Battle of the Bands competition had previously published the results in the local Gazette and Evening News so everyone knew of Seachimp by now. They were praised heartily and received a Mayor's congratulations in the paper. Their recording contract meant that they would be welcome to tour first, then record next in the local recording studio. Claire was very excited about the prospect of going up in the world in this way.

HMV had agreed to allow Seachimp to do a day's disc signing in the store once the album was released. They were expecting a lot of fans to step forwards to make a purchase in this way. Advertising was plenty and the band had often played in Collage, so killing two birds with one stone, so to speak.

Alex Davies took delight in the band's progress. He knew Claire's story, her personal struggles and traumas. He had seen the band play so many times in his own restaurant and been witness to this latest coup of musical achievement. Alex was an entrepreneur, no mistaking that one, and to see his 'own people' succeed in their respective fields was definitely on the cards. He warmed to the fact, and felt involved; responsible in his own way for Seachimp's success.

What would they call the album? Claire was no good with names, so figured that that detail ought to be left until the band had clubbed together in the studio. Signed to record a twelve song album, the compilation was due for release within a six-week period.

So Charlie and Claire, parents-to-be; business, music, family. How would this all tie in together? Would it be possible at all? Curiously, they were asking less between the two of them and working more on solutions. Charlie had a cracking theory that 'if desired, the solution will always present itself – every time!' Claire had, at first hearing, told him how arrogant that sounded, then gradually grown to appreciate the optimistic connotations that such a statement alluded to.

Anyway, they were pretty much fixed up by now, so what would remain would be to ensure a secure beginning for Morris jr. Would the albums sell well enough? Would the tropical fish be desired? Would business thrive (as intended), or would reality turn and smack these two back in the face all over again?

Charlie Morris was going to marry Claire Halls. They were going to have a baby together, and in the mean time record an album and run a tropical fish store in town. Surely this would be enough to keep any person occupied and out of trouble. Surely the goose would not become a gander. Surely these two could fly high on the wings of paradise together. After all they deserved the best, now that they had come through their rough patches simultaneously.

"Breathe me, Charlie Morris" Claire whispered in his ear as he left for work on a Monday morning.

"You're my angel," he replied simply.

They were psychologically tied. Involved with each other to the core, something big was on the horizon. Like chasing a rainbow, there would be little point in moving any faster in order to try to catch the pot of gold. The future remained that bit too distant to grasp outright. Always moving, always grooving, these folk had their eyes set ahead of the game now.

Coming from where they had just been, it seemed all the more miraculous. But, they were making themselves and busy in the process too. They had support, they had friends, they had gigs lined up and custom to deliver towards. They had responsibilities and affects to look after.

Ben Williams played no role really in the line of Seachimp or their relationship. Only, as he was part of the crew he had of course learnt the news via Tim Richardson. He made an exception to his usual routine and picked up the phone to call Charlie:

"Hi! Charlie? It's Ben Williams here".

"Oh, right, OK, how's things? What's up?"

"I just called to congratulate you and Claire on your engagement. I wanted to wish you both well and much health, prosperity, and good things."

"That's very kind of you Ben – thankyou very much indeed."

"I sent a card in the post yesterday so it should be with you by tomorrow at the latest."

"That's great. I really appreciate your calling now. Cheers!"

"No problem. Feel free to call if you want. I'm going to see Tim tomorrow morning as he is training on the course. I have some advice for him."

"Fair enough. See you soon."

"Yes, great. Bye."

That was a rare phone call indeed, as they usually met at Collage as part of the crew. Sometimes they might bump into each other on the street when Ben would walk his Cocker Spaniel in the afternoon, although he preferred to find some countryside for the dog walks.

Charlie's spirits lifted as a consequence. He got on with the day's work and received a couple of orders for an aquarium in someone's living room, and one in a restaurant reception. Surprising how popular the tropical fish could be. They were in demand all over the county in fact, so some days he would be just driving to deliver a tank and fish. The van was an opal green Vauxhall.

Claire took herself off for a long walk along the disused railway track. She ended up at the Hayburn Wyke pub on the coast after a two hour walk. She ordered a light lunch, soup, bread rolls and a coca-cola, then walked back once again. She probably did this to keep fit and slim without having to go to the gym, or run, or swim vigorously. It worked. A four hour afternoon walk on a quiet day tired her out and she called in Fish4U! before crashing out with a mug of cocoa.

No day would ever again be a dull day.

Chapter 8
The Flaming Squirrels

Alex had decided. It was time to expand his business repertoire. He was going to open up a coffee shop as well.

Suzanna had been expressing an interest right from the early days of conception. That is, conception of a proposed business idea.

So they were both up for this. Melanie, Alex's wife, and Fiona – their daughter – would both be involved with the decision making and maintenance of the workplace. The decision was not one to be taken lightly, or be made nonchalantly.

The idea came from Suzanna Jeffries. 'What to call the café?'

She had suggested '*The Flaming Squirrels*' on account of an early morning vision that she had encountered on a continental bus trip. She had been sat on the bus in an awake state and been absently looking out of the window. As the bus traversed a bridge the lights reflected off the struts in such a way that the bus's movement made it look like a group of flaming squirrels running across the bridge. She had been profoundly impressed by this encounter.

The impression had stuck with her and as a commemoration to the event thought that the café ought to be called 'The Flaming Squirrels'. Alex's curiosity was aroused but no other name could match that for both originality and appeal.

So, in this way the name was elected and they were able to move onto the next stage of development. This would be a family run enterprise and Miss Jeffries would be an accepted member of the Davies' empire. She would be Assistant Manager in fact. Alex had been relying on her in Collage for the past two years and she had proved a remarkable colleague, always careful, astute, and honest to work with.

With this in mind and impressed by her dedication to Triathlon, Alex had decided to hire her in a more responsible position as of now.

Would this affect the way things stood already? Would there be any digressions? Would there be in-fighting over a position of authority? That would remain to be seen and only time would tell.

Probably, their personal niggles would be manageable. As there had been no major kerfuffles within Collage there was a sense of trust, telepathy and destiny amongst them. Alex was aware that the competition amongst local cafes was already high. He would have to bring the café into an immaculate shape in a very sort period of time in order to compete and stay alive. Would this challenge be unattainable? Or would The Flaming Squirrels thrive amongst the others? Alex Davies was determined that the latter should be the case.

Having ran the restaurant for years by now, and worked in the trade since leaving school aged 16, Alex was quietly confident that things would work out for the best. Although not exactly literally the quiet, shy type, he was optimistic that his ideas would make the transition from new concept to regular enterprise.

Melanie was busy as mother and artist, Fiona was at grade school, and Alex was dad, manager, entrepreneur. He had a flare for life, a certain joie de vivre that people were ready to acknowledge on a regular basis by coming to eat at Collage.

So, a café-sandwich bar, or a coffee shop offering unique blends of coffee and other assorted beverages. Whatever would be deemed the best outcome would be created. There were funds available from Collage and from an enterprise scheme. He had considered applying to the Lottery Guild as well, but figured that he should make do with what he already had.

"The Flaming Squirrels – yes, I like that," uttered Alex; "The place to hang out, to enjoy a quiet cup of coffee, tea, or a smoothie. The place to be."

He had begun to rub his hands together in mercenary glee as the thought sunk home in his mind.

"Not just any old café, not your ordinary establishment, but a place of authenticity. A place to soak up some cultural rays. The place to become a complete person." He began to fantasise for a moment about the success that would surely come.

He was uncharacteristically like this. Usually, Alex was a pragmatist, a very hands-on, nose to the grind stone type of operator. But for once he had allowed his mind to wander towards the future prospects that lay ahead.

So, between them all they were very excited and looking forwards to the grand opening. He had £35,000 to open up shop with and the premises had been located at a relatively near-by spot.

There were thoughts of holding music and poetry evenings at the café; Cabaret too. It would be ideally a central point of local cultural significance for people to visit and appreciate on a regular basis. He had taken into account the cut-throat nature of the world of commerce and was preparing to deal with the competition.

This was actually something that worried Alex slightly. Generally speaking he was unshakeable, but the prospect of conflict and the possibility of unrest concerned him. He had every intention of focusing his energies on the task at hand, and no real intention of having his affairs muddied over by intruders, bystanders, or interferers. This however could never be guaranteed.

As is the case with any project, set-backs were to be expected, the status quo to be shaken in some way, the apple cart to be slightly upset (which nobody ever liked particularly), or the boat to be rocked. So long as his ship didn't sink he would be a happy man. So long as his hard work and perseverance continued to pay off he would be legitimately affluent. He wouldn't mind so long as Collage and the café were fully functional and the family intact.

Melanie understood all this. She knew how much it meant to Alex to be in control of his life and affairs. He wore the trousers in the Davies' household, very much. However, that is not to say that everyone else took a back seat. Far from it. The Davies were all encouraged by one another to take a driver's seat. Even Fiona was already a real character at her young age. The kids at playschool got on with her and she had lots of friends. Lots of energy and a bundle of laughs, she looked promising as a future heir to the Davies' hospitality regime.

Alex had done some research with his wife, interviewing over one hundred coffee shop/café owners in the space of two years. Having compiled the data they had decided that the following criteria were necessary for running a successful establishment.

Each hired barista should demonstrate a passion for coffee, the ability to work quickly and logically whilst working on their feet to a professional standard. Physical fitness should prove adequate for the job especially because the job would be demanding and require a lot of movement. A barista should be able to multi-task – taking orders, making the order up, arithmetic for calculating costs, waiting on the tables, cleaning up after and holding some friendly banter in the interim.

Suzanna had already demonstrated an insider knowledge of the trade...suppliers, labour laws, tax regimes and Fairtrade. She knew how to operate technical instruments as well, so made the ideal employee. Alex had calculated that he would require five staff on part-time basis to run the show. He had already taken into account the local availability of trades personnel – plumbing, carpenter, electrician, decorator – to step in when needed.

The practical layout of the café would be another question in hand. To be accessible for wheelchairs, to serve organic, vegetarian, vegan, and gluten-free products; to cater for the young and the elderly, eg teacakes for some, milkshakes for others. There would be maximum consideration of health and hygiene, personal cleanliness and general germ-free maintenance of the preparation areas.

Alex had considered buying bean bags, a sofa, and some comfortable armchairs to place in the room. Contemplating the décor, the artwork, he had spoken to Melanie. And regarding a tropical fish tank, he of course had phoned Charlie Morris.

"Don't copy others, stick to what you are good at. Create your own niche and stick at it…..do not reinvent the wheel!" one café owner had advised him upon enquiring.

"We look at our service – how we can give a better service, ways to speed up the service but be friendly. Always forward thinking – about what else we can offer the customer", another independent café had mentioned.

Alex knew what qualities he was looking for in his staff. He would especially look out for customer-oriented, friendly disposition, sense of humour, communicable and diplomatic. He wanted to hire people who paid attention to small details and made an effort to remember people's names and circumstances if they were regulars. Those who showed persistence would get the job. Suzanna already passed the test through working at Collage.

One wise speculator had told Alex "consolidate on what you do best; get quality, quantity and price correct and then cross your fingers".

One more important quality that Alex was looking out for was reliability with finances. Somebody who could demonstrate an ability for correct, efficient arithmetic and astute accounting skills would get the job.

Melanie had advised him to always think 'What else can you offer the customer? What situations should you anticipate and prepare for?' He knew that a lot more thinking would have to be done here. There was no intention of opening an internet café however. He thought more a music café if anything.

The weaknesses, both potential and actual that he had taken into account included lack of ownership experience in this field. Hence the need for a team. He was worried about a lack of client base. What would happen if nobody showed up to eat and drink here? If somebody showed up for a day's work looking dishevelled and shabby, tired and flat in character, what on earth would he do? Possibly send them home again with a severe warning not to do it again.

He hoped to hire workers who got on, where personal conflicts would not disturb the work ethic. None if at all possible. If somebody became selfish thinking only 'what is in this for me?' then a point would be raised, of course. The idea was to provide a service to the local community, to be a significant contributor, to enable people to eat, drink and be merry in the establishment.

The café would be a non-smoking venue. Prohibited within the building. Would the logistics of this venture work out? Would there be sufficient income? Would he pay off his loans and make a profit? Alex held a philosophy that a weakness was only a weakness if one viewed failure as an end in itself, rather than a stepping stone towards newer successful means. He held the notion that to build a credible reputation from scratch would involve initiative, contribution, and customer interest. The latter would sort itself out, he hoped.

As far as publicity and marketing were concerned he was prepared to talk to the local media and put some adverts in the papers and on the radio, in magazines and 'What's On' guides. Other cafes would hopefully pass the message on by word of mouth. What was his target market? Well, in truth, he decided to aim for all – young, old, male, female, student, and professional. He hoped that any 'business angels' might lend a hand if in favour of the project.

What threats there were would surely be from the existing venues, the chains, the big-name stores, the firm and steadfast. He had thought about flooding, electrical faults, woodworm, diseases, graffiti, and broken windows too. These could be potential obstacles to overcome.

The trouble would be, what if Costa Coffee, Starbucks or Café Nero got all the attention? There must surely be those who prefer an independent branch coffee house? If so, if they found him and The Flaming Squirrels then all would be well.

Alex knew in his heart of hearts that the only certainty is in fact uncertainty. The risk would be a gamble, but one which he and the team were prepared to make. With his £35,000 he could make a decent start. He would stand a fair chance of winning in his field still.

He and Suzanna had decided that *The Flaming Squirrels* would support both Fair Trade and Organic products. This would give the farmers incentive to continue growing coffee beans in South/Central America. He recognised that small businesses, his included, were the life-blood of the local community.

They had agreed on a five-year plan. In this time, all debts were to be paid off. The timescale was sufficient for them and all the world to know whether or not the café would flourish or flounder. So long as they were breaking even in this time all would be well.

How specific would he need to be to set-up shop? Well, he and the 'team' had always been as hawk-eyed as possible, and continued to expect to be so. There were to be five stages of venture assimilation between conception and realisation.

1) Research and information collection
2) Information assimilation and financial projections
3) Application of theory into practice
4) Marketing the said enterprise to gain good custom
5) Appraisal of how successful the operation would run

Would they thrive and survive, sink, swim, or be forced to reevaluate? Time would surely tell. Alex had always been a wise guy, making sure that his lean times could enable preparation for better times to come.

Alex had made it clear that the philosophy of the café would involve interpersonal concordance and reciprocal role-taking. In this way a collaboration would enable efficient operations to occur, essential for an unfolding scheme.

Up until this time, any invective at Collage had been dealt with swiftly and professionally by Alex. He had been master of the art of dealing with neurotic customers. Master of ceremonies.

Claire and Charlie were, from time to time, consulted on the matter. There may still have been traces of a problematic period for her, as she tended to smoke when stressed out. Cigarettes, or roll-up tobacco were her norms of procedure. And when she smoked she felt free, as did Charlie when he joined in. They both didn't mind an occasional smoke, although they respected the rules of the cafeteria when entering for some nourishment. That was, no-smoking within the establishment.

Claire was still coming to terms with the news of her friend Megan, and the death of her husband Henry. It had really sunk in now and got to her most inner being. Megan had been scarred by this loss and their son Darren too. He had lost his father and been told he had gone on vacation. There was to be no real compensation for these events. By talking to Charlie about it, Claire could learn to come to terms with this. The crew were listening in.

"I read the news last week. Something awful has happened. My best friend from college, Megan, she got married. That's not the awful news though. Her husband Henry got killed. One of her previous liaisons came back with a vengeance. They knew who had done it and eventually caught him in Portugal."

"Bloody hell Claire, what would drive someone to kill a man?" Charlie asked angrily.

"They said he was jealous and emotion got the better of him after Megan and Henry got hitched. They identified him as Robert Dodsworth. Megan used to call him Robbie when they were together."

"Damn it Claire, why can't a man just move on and accept what is over is over. There's no point flogging a dead horse."

"Robbie had become obsessive and used to hang around their house on an evening. He had been warned already but took no notice. After he had done it Megan was left scared with her young son in her arms. Robbie fled and she called the cops. Henry was in the living room at the time of intrusion, tried to defend himself but got stabbed in the chest. Oh God, I can't take this." Claire burst into tears.

Charlie put an arm around her and sat there solemnly for a while. Then he asked "How did they get onto him in Portugal?"

"He left the country the same day by car, and caught the ferry onto the continent. The car was spotted several times in Holland, France, Spain and then eventually Portugal where he was arrested. His home in England got raided. That's where they found the car registration details and made an international alert. The search took three months though. There was a huge car chase with patrols on the ground and helicopters in the air."

"So they had i.d., motives and Megan's testimony. What a twisted mind to actually do that."

"When he was caught all he talked about was some woman he had an affair with on the run. He reckoned that she was carrying his child. Sick bastard."

"What about Megan and her little boy though. Where did they go while all this was going on?"

"They were taken into shelter until the arrest was confirmed. She was mortified and little Darren didn't know where his daddy had gone."

"So in his twisted little mind he figured that by killing her husband, Megan would have more room for him again. What a waste. Henry Belvedere, what a promising future together just blown away by some moronic intervention. Makes me sick to think about it."

"She even thought about going to visit him to see what he had to say. He was just chasing rainbows the whole time. No matter how close you get they just keep on moving away."

They both sat there silently mulling the news over, whilst the rest of the crew took a back seat and wondered.

Alex had learnt of their news as well. He sympathised but felt relieved that they still respected his rules. He felt honoured. To have friends like these could only be a good thing. How would these two fit in with The Flaming Squirrels? They would be welcome guests at all times, an invite with an open door and classed as prime customers. They would never work for Alex as Suzanna would and did already, but they had a regular place within the 'crew'.

As for smoking, there would be none within Davies hospitality inc, but Charlie knew there were many reasons within reasons from Fish4U! already so as not to pollute the atmosphere within the area.

Charlie never used to smoke and picked up the occasional cigarette as a direct result of Claire's behaviour. In effect he had picked it up out of osmosis, and the stress that he felt meant that a way out was necessary from time to time, or as the Spanish would say, 'de vez en cuando.'

They were a cosmopolitan bunch here. That could only be a good thing for setting up a catering company. With visits to France, Denmark, Spain and other continental locations there were already allusions towards a multi-ethnic cuisine being presented within the café and at Collage. The idea, it seemed, would appeal to a broader audience back home in Scarborough. At least that was the plan of action intended.

Interruptions affected Alex all the time. He was made of stout stuff, solid material so would be able to deal with these in his own way. The others were also affected by interruptions as well. Sometimes they would really, truly peeve Charlie off. So much so that an inspired move by the grace of God, on becoming interrupted by some nagging pestilent beings became either obsolete or otherwise completely off the track of where it should have been going to.

He was ultimately agitated by these uncanny interruptions that so rudely distracted him from his work and creative direction. Claire would occasionally be interrupted half way through a song or piece of music and this would make her feel like killing somebody dead as they stood. In truth it was just as well that a guitar would be in hand. "Nothing so rude as an ignorant disturbance," they agreed.

On becoming stressed out what do you do? Do you continue as before with the project at hand? Does one drop the dead donkey and scream blue murder to high heaven? Do you step outside, get out a cigarette and smoke it? Or should one pretend that all is well and drink yet another cup of toxic caffeine in a mug and self-destruct in a perfectly legal manner?

If the answer was 'none of the above', then please drop your solution on a feedback form to Alex Davies at *The Flaming Squirrels* and you would be gratefully thanked for your important contribution to the café's development. What is more, for the most original feedback of the month there would be a free drink and something to eat every once in a while so all comers would be welcome to comment.

"I hate myself better than you so come on over and don't be blue, let it all hang out, let it all hang out, let it shine, let it all hang out, yeah!" said Claire one afternoon feeling a wee bit moody, to Charlie Morris.

"Well ain't that just a great thing, sweetheart? Best not lose sleep over it anyway. What's up? What's got to you?" he replied with an ear open.

"Can't you see that it's just not the same anymore. Life just never stays the frickin' same. Why can't the good days last forever? Tell me that O oracle," she asked.

"You know what, C? We all have the same 24 hours 7 days a week. Maybe somehow we just have to get on with it and see what comes out every day. Who knows, you may get something good for your troubles," he said.

"Gee, thanks mate. If only Seachimp would comply with that then we would be truly sorted. It's a calamity you know. A catastrophe, a trial and a trauma. We're doomed, all doomed!"

"Whoa! Steady on there, easy girl, don't be too hard on yourself. You know already what you can do, and what is more, there are others who appreciate your stuff already. Keep at it, keep truckin', keep plugging away. Don't be so hard on yourself," Charlie advised.

They went into a silent mode for half an hour before anything else was said, as though there was something of import to be thinking about. And then she looked at him intensely for 10 seconds and smiled a big grin.

"You're right. Again! I should keep at it and plough on. Nobody is going to plough my furrows for me. The farmer must drive his oxen. And I must drive the band. You're right and I want to thank you for that." Claire broke the silence.

Charlie simply acknowledged this with a smile and hugged her.

The day was far from over and plans were being devised for the cafeteria. So back to Alex Davies and Suzanna Jeffries. Their plans were about to be processed and put into action. The baby was being born, so to speak. The Flaming Squirrels was a-go-go. The plan was in action.

They had plenty of experience and research evidence between them by now, and that was all going to fit into the grander scheme of things. The way things were due to work, the manner in which the operations would run, the mechanism of the whole, the grease to the cogs of the machinery, the spark to the flame. All was in order by this time. And what is more, they were revelling in the prospects, too.

Suzanna frequently got a sensation in her stomach as though there were butterflies taking flight within. She put this down to the fact that she was a key player and would never allow this sensation to dominate her like a silverback gorilla. She was in control and about to take it all to a whole new level.

The fact that this was a supported cause meant that it was real. The operation would really unfold and take place. It was going to occur in practical, actual reality; the café, the crew, the team, the people, the business, the functioning of a valid hospitality unit in town on a daily basis. This meant so much to her that she would get rather possessive and defensive if somebody were to utter any words against it.

Being jealously possessive had its problems. For one, she may have got a blinkered view of what else was going on around and about. Although she had Tim and Shane, her brother, to keep her on track, when determinedly focused on the enterprise things got a little exciting from time to time.

When peeved off at another person there would be no real argument, more a subtle shift of character and vocal intonation as if to say 'there we go, I'm right as per usual; so hear me through' kind of thing.

Anyway, the point here was *The Flaming Squirrels* and the opening day. It came round in June 2013. An early summer-time opening. They were all there, Alex Davies, Suzanna Jeffries, Melanie, Fiona, Shane, Charlie Morris, Claire Halls, Ben Williams, Tim Richardson. The crew turned up on opening day at various times to support the new enterprise. Along with fifty other new customers who had seen the opening day advertised in the Evening Mail or by Yorkshire Coast Radio. They were in for the new experience and to show willing to support a good proprietor and a quality chef.

Alex was delighted to be selected as 'New Venture of the Month' in the local news. Plenty of other bar owners/restaurateurs/ baristas had decided to show up with words of advice and encouragement, or some with a more competitive slant declaring how hard it would be to so much as survive in the environment. He knew that within a five year period approximately 85% of small businesses went bankrupt and fell through. With this in mind he felt determined to be one of the 15% who succeeded.

So *The Flaming Squirrels* was happening. No longer a hypothetical thought in two people's minds. It was a –go, all stops pulled out and sailing over the horizon blue; Day one and plenty of good custom to see it through.

"You know, the thing with a new café is to keep it all fresh. Even the tiles on the wall have to sparkle," one man offered.

"You need to cater to an ever-changing and divergent sense of customer taste," one lady explained.

"Never mind keeping up with the Jones's, you must create your own style and unique brand to attract a niche market," said another.

The comments came in all day and Alex was really chuffed to bits that people would bother to contribute to his cause in this way. He realised that he was facing an uphill struggle along the way and needed to prepare not only his body and mind for the challenge, but also that of his staff, and the groundwork for the café would need to be regularly evaluated as well.

Fortunately there were no bricks through windows on day one, and the crew had decided that the leftover edibles should be given to the homeless 'Shelter' charity in the local area. This would at least add a bit of credibility to the place. As well as which, this act would count in favour of social conscience on their behalf.

There were at least a dozen other local cafes to compete with and Alex had spoken with owners of the following establishments already prior to setting up shop: Roasters coffee shop (fresh coffee specialists), Café Heart (salad impresarios), café Baroque (nice French patio theme going on), Tummy Busters (great for a full English cooked breakfast), Café Rendezvous (smokey meeting place for all comers), Mr Milo's (an upstairs, modern, artsy joint), Boddy's (two modern art deco establishments) and so many others too.

Anyhow, there it all is; *The Flaming Squirrels*, the owner, the staff, and all the people. An improved state of affairs. After a long time of deliberation, contemplation and otherwise procrastination, Alex Davies finally owned two establishments in Scarborough. He was a businessman and respected by the local community.

Tim had been training that morning and decided to spend his lunch break at the café. He arrived and immediately felt impressed.

"Man, this is totally a welcome break from that jive you know," as he had been busy at the training session which had just elapsed. He had been swimming as usual on the morning schedule.

"Hmmmm, you could say that you are a welcome break from the grind too," replied Alex.

"Thanks", uttered Tim. "May I see the menu, please?"

"Sure thing," Alex clapped his hands twice in an authoritarian manner and Dani the new barista brought a menu over to the table. There were already items on the blackboard, but he was keen to incorporate a more personal touch for Tim on the first day.

"Thankyou…I would like a fruits of the forest smoothie and a tuna and cucumber ciabatta, please".

"Very well. Bear with me just five minutes and it will be yours sir," Alex declared.

Five minutes passed and sure enough, Tim was given his lunch. As a special offer, the first one thousand customers were being given a complementary wrist band to take away with them promoting The Flaming Squirrels. Hopefully they would be worn and the person would return to eat there at some point.

"My father would be impressed with your café, Alex", Tim told him. He knew this for a fact as his dad was something of a gourmandiser at the best of times. Alex grinned impishly at the prospect of such a compliment.

"Thanks buddy. It's always good to hear such a thing in truth." Alex grinned even more openly now.

'Let the celebrations commence.' The café was rolling, Collage was rolling, the punters were rolling, the commerce was rolling, all was rolling. Their tragic moments had been forgotten about in the face of a new lease of life here at The Flaming Squirrels. All was not lost after all.

Far from it in fact. Ben had brought Pépé along as well and promptly sat outside, on the patio with his four-legged friend. This was permissible, however; just no dogs inside the building. "Shucks," thought Ben, but he was far from complaining anyway.

Ben ordered a cappuccino with blueberry muffin. He was given a large mug and a large bun. This suited him just fine anyway as he was hungry by now. He sat there sufficiently contented for half an hour, all the while talking to Pépé and attempting to attract the attention of Suzanna between jobs. She was busy on her feet the whole day and was fully aware of Benjamin's ploy. It was all quite a lot of fun, truth being told.

Ben was known for being a bit eccentric by now, but his relationship as mentor with Tim had really been a key focal point as it developed. Ben was a clever man, but just had an inferiority complex as far as the Jeffries' were concerned. Shane had determinedly fixed him with the fear of God for no good reason. He was a bit of a bastard at times, was Shane. A bit loopy, a wee bit unpredictable, and all in the name of science.

Shane considered that his 'experiments' were all in the cause of advancing science. Some would agree, some would put it down to a more rebellious urge to annihilate those he didn't care for. Ben, for example, seemed to be standing in his way, permanently. Shane was the only player to even think of it in this way; Suzanna represented a chance, an opportunity, an inkling of interest. Ben may one day have his own way, but for now he would have to stick with the university job and looking after the dog.

He was essentially a responsible character. This was a good thing. Ben left the café at 2pm and went on his way. Shortly after 3pm Charlie and Claire turned up for the 'grand opening' day. They sat indoors. Although neither felt like eating anything on this occasion, they shared a pot of tea and told Alex how impressed they were with his new venture. He had made a courageous step, everybody agreed.

Shane came round to see his sister and give her an update on the day's activities (of which there were not a great deal). There was a lot more happening here at The Flaming Squirrels, after all. He ordered a fruit juice (orange with ice), an egg mayonnaise and avocado sandwich, and sat in for twenty minutes eating, drinking and being imperturbably impressed in his own way.

At least they all knew where they stood. "Time for a cigarette," Claire announced to Charlie. And with that she unrolled a packet of Golden Virginia tobacco and a king-size rizla paper, and proceeded to roll up a smoke. She went outside and lit it. Smoking contentedly for five minutes, she proceeded to admire the passers-by and thought for a moment how her role in Seachimp could expand now that this café was rolling. It was, after all, due to become a music and poetry café on an evening. As well as being a hangout for local artists to display their work, Seachimp could give a gig or two there once in a while, she figured.

The early days for The Flaming Squirrels were due to be café only. Alex was working on the music licensing procedure. It was to be a coup for a later date, no doubt. No music, no art, no punters, he thought. Probably correctly, mind. Everyone liked a bit of entertainment occasionally.

The Flaming Squirrels was to be a place for all. Still, again, yet to be, always was, will be someday....you name it and this place would speak it, whether in product, quality, or flare for originality. A cool café, where you may even see the Pink Panther were you to look close enough.

So that would be the story for how it actually opened, from conception to realisation within a three year period. 'With a little help from my friends' was the theme tune on opening day, along with some Stevie Wonder/Dionne Warwick 'That's what friends are for', and some other boogie music, The Flaming Squirrels café came into being.

The question arose, who would have the honour of opening music night? Would it be Seachimp? Or would it be otherwise? The first month would be music-free, following which Alex had decided to invite some local musicians like Jesse Hutchinson, Carl Woodford, or Amalya Huntley to the spot.

Would The Flaming Squirrels survive? Well, with a lineup like that, one can only imagine that this ship would sail. Sailing on the oceans blue, where the waves were high and the crew caused a to-do. Sailing in Scar-the-borough on the streets, where the atmosphere was right and the people liked to meet.

They were full of ditties like this and at least they were put to work...into action, front line duty boys and girls. Café time!

Chapter 9
The Seachimp Tour

Seachimp had been offered a UK tour playing pubs and clubs. Charlie had offered to be the driver, the road manager. The band were given over fifteen gigs in a three week period in Scotland, Wales and England. Due to travel up to Glasgow, The Isle of Skye, Inverness, Aberdeen and Edinburgh, then South down the West coast to Liverpool via Carlisle, Manchester, Cardiff, Bristol and Birmingham; Seachimp were excited. Coming back home via the Midlands, then back to Yorkshire.

It didn't make it easy that Claire was already two and a half months pregnant with Charlie's baby. She was keen to make it work, anyhow, simultaneously desiring her own child, and committing responsibility to the band at this crucial time in its early development. She figured that there was time to squeeze in a tour before the big day arrived, though.

Charlie had decided to act as road manager, hiring out the 16- seater minibus for the band members and all their equipment. He wanted, and had their consent, to drive them round and act as chauffeur in order to play a key role for the band. After all, he had seen the whole thing come into play over the last 18 months in local venues, and their recording contract seemed to be working. Heads were taking note. Records were selling and phone calls kept coming in with various offers of one kind or another.

Whether a photo shoot, a magazine article, or an e-zine for the web page to connect, Seachimp were coming on.

"Well, you know what, Charlie? If you don't grab hold, you would be alone. We don't want that," Claire told him during the arrangements time.

"I don't intend to catch the heebie-jeebies, you know, C" he mentioned back to her.

"Somebody told me that to learn your limits you have to exceed them in the first place," Claire continued.

"It's almost as if I know where I'm going but I've forgotten how to get there," he mused.

"Well, silly, here's the itinerary," and she slapped the note down on the table in front of his face.

Random acts of kindness such as this were few and far between for these two. They never particularly squabbled, although Claire would have been doing her utmost on occasion to instigate such an event. Charlie refused to be drawn in and often cogitated instead. Many a potential argument had blown over because of his defensive mechanism. Maybe he was just scared of losing her, that's all.

"Gotta look after the human spirit," a great A1 sized poster instructed from the wall of their bedroom.

Maybe it was ironic that this was precisely the element of life that had previously caused Claire so much suffering. That is, until Charlie had swept her up in such style.

Somedays Claire would tell a despondent Charlie, "Take your fed-uppity elsewhere, big boy," or simply, "Hang loose – you never know where you might end up".

And Charlie would reply "Who gives a farooq?" feeling blue and moody.

Moments of tension cropped up every now and again, especially as they were attempting to fathom the untold responsibility that would come upon them within the next 12 months. Whereas she desired to settle down and get a grip, Charlie was still a little reluctant to settle into fatherhood and mature, paternal responsibility.

"Half the time we're going, we don't know why or where," he told Claire one day.

"Oh crikes, you're beginning to sound like Ozzy Osbourne! Get a grip, man".

Charlie farted out loud.

"Oi – thunderpants Kaplinsky – behave!" she raised her voice.

Sometimes they would invent names for each other to pass the time of day. Claire was lauded with titles such as Little Miss Spendapenny, Chuckalooby Stroodlepants, Wanda Basaconda, or it could even stretch to The Funky Monkey, Ellity Verriot, or Saturday Night Beaver.

In return he would find himself bestowed with nick-names such as Prometheus von Vofflecronk, Okbagula Rundthunk, Melifluous Mr T, Corporal Matey, or Tight-pants Malone. Or on occasion, Bilge-pump Charlie, Alfonso Clutterbucket, or Captain Spliffy. Both had previously smoked an occasional joint, but had cooled off for quite some time now, preferring to stick to the odd cigarette here and there.

The South-Central American Miss Anacon Menendez would also feature, as would the Chinese lady Y'Un Tao Ping, or the American homecoming Queen Busty Winkleman. They certainly had a barrel of laughs coming up with the new honours list every now and again.

Once she caught him reading an extract from the book of Romans in the Bible. "Whatever is becoming of you? You shall be now known as the Right Reverend Hastings Barbanwadiboo, and long may it last," she warned.

Charlie only half paid attention to this nonsense and carried right on reading about how the potter has the right to mould the clay in whatever fashion he so chooses, just as teachers have the right to shape their pupils' minds as demands the curriculum. In the same way, night followed day followed night followed day; and so on and so forth.

"Charlie, do you think that Seachimp is the right name for our band? What would happen if we changed our name?"

"What have you got in mind?" he asked her.

"I had a brainwave, a flash of brilliance – what if our band was called 'Umbilicus'?"

"Umbilicus, eh? Hmmmm well that is a good name for a band, I must admit. Trouble is, C, it may confuse the punters. They will all want to hear Seachimp. After all, they have already bought the records!" Charlie offered in response.

"Sensible answer, Mr T", she said and finalised the conversation.

They went on preparing for quite some time, and making calls to other band members meanwhile. The tour was due to depart in two weeks time, so there was plenty of time for adjustment and learning the itinerary as well.

Claire had been considering incorporating a violin player into the group for a few of their tracks. Being a folk-rock band there were many, many potential avenues for including new instruments every now and again.

So there they were, and going to stick with the original line-up and keep the band's name as well. "We don't want any further confusions now, do we Charlie?" Claire muttered.

Although, their producer had hinted that some new sounds would improve record sales, the band still had an awful long way to go before they hit the big time. So they would make do with a UK tour (of smaller venues) and a steady stream of record sales to boot.

The time was fast approaching for take-off. No more Groundhog days now. Things were moving on and at a rapid rate of knots to say the least. Claire was internally anxious about her developing foetus, and had been given the all-clear to carry on singing for a few months more before totally resting up.

She would make subtle remarks to Charlie which sometimes were like water off a duck's back, neither sinking in nor making anything of an impact on him. 'Typical bloke,' she thought. Anyway, he was doing a great favour now and honouring the band as driver for the three week duration. Probably also a bit of the old MC work from time to time, and an element of security as well. So a good guy to have around.

One week to go and the plans all came together, last minute rehearsals and then the day came for departure. They were due to travel about in a 16-seater minibus rented from Enterprise Vehicles for a month's duration. They had decided to do some sight-seeing in between times as well.

So, first stop Glasgow. The group set off at 8.30am that morning and arrived in plenty of time. Their main fear was being involved with any form of local aggression. Being once the European Capital City of Culture, this would be a highlight and a first gig. Once in town, by 5.30pm, they went and found their digs first and unloaded some baggage.

After a trip to the local pizzeria, the band made their way to their venue for the night and set up shop in the bar 'The Highlander'. Not a huge place, but set to seat well over 100 punters at capacity, the ambience was right for the night.

At the mic at 9pm Charlie stood up and announced "Ladies and Gentlemen, all the way from Scarborough, Yorkshire, I am proud to present to you tonight a band which offers folk, blues and rock; please give a warm welcome to 'Seachimp'!"

The room rocked for a moment with whistles and applause, then off they went with their first set. Their were some real characters present that night, dressed up in contemporary gear with shirts, jackets, trousers, and shoes. Women in flirty and revealing attire, men in bombastic macho denim, leather or otherwise attractive wear.

Claire totally rocked the house on that first night. There were no indications of travel fatigue, and no in-fighting amongst the colleagues. Charlie looked around the room and saw people having a good time. He was pleased at that.

The night went well, and by 11.30pm Seachimp had officially played Glasgow. 12 CDs sold at the desk, making a tidy sum of

£144 from that area, plus tickets at the door at £3/head. So a total sum of £444 from that one night.

The band returned to their hotel exhausted and everyone had a quick celebration before focusing their efforts on the tour ahead. Next stop Isle of Skye – notoriously awkward driving, narrow lanes and an awful lot of country-seaside views. So how long would it take them to locate the township and their location to gig?

The day began well – everyone got out of bed. Breakfast in the restaurant, and bags packed, then away they went. Charlie carefully monitored the practical timing of the travelling, ensuring that everyone was ready and on time for the next move before setting off.

They left Glasgow by 10am and set off travelling to The Isle of Skye, figuring to call in the Talisker Whisky distillery en route. Well, technically, it was way off route, but they had the time. Then the weather turned sour and it began to rain as they travelled. Not just itsy-bitsy rain, but sporadic deluges, washing the windows as they drove.

In a nutshell, just less than half the proceeds from The Highlander the night before went on bottles of Scottish Malt Whiskey, some as mature as 30 years. They figured that it would count as a souvenir if nothing else. "The delights of the amber nectar," proclaimed the drummer as they drove on.

They found the pub in a small town, but sure enough there was a crowd for the band. Maybe forty-five people had turned out on this night to see them at £4/head, so £180 in takings on this occasion. They each wondered how that would be spent over the next week.

The gig seemed to liven up a quiet, sleepy old town and some of the locals were dancing away to the sound of the music, really having an enjoyable time and experiencing the fine sounds of Seachimp. There was no trouble and Charlie did not need to step into any untoward turbulences on The Isle of Skye. He was blessed. They all were blessed.

The band hung around the pub until closing time at one o'clock a.m. Claire got talking to a group of local fishermen who spun their yarns of yore and folklore. They all were rapt in the unravellings of the night.

That night they stayed in a Bed and Breakfast farmhouse. The van was parked up outside and the rain could be heard bouncing off the roof during the early hours of the morning. Rising at 8 am with a sense of anticipation for the forthcoming trip they were ready and off by 10a.m. once again, leaving their gratitude with the inn keeper and farmhouse owner.

"Let's stop of at Loch Ness for a swim today," suggested Claire as they drove towards Inverness. She had a crazy notion to swim in the water when they arrived.

"Are ye nae afraid of Nessie, the monster from the deep, lassie?" the drummer joked in a Scottish accent.

"Don't be silly, Pete – it'll be a laugh," she retorted.

The group meditated on the kind of laugh they were about to experience that day, then Dan felt glad to have brought his camcorder... "I'll stay by the bankside filming – you'se guys can all go in the water, though".

"Chicken – chck, chck, chck, chck," they intoned back at him.

They laughed for a while then the new day began for all of them, and off they travelled once again to Inverness round by the top of the Grampians, to the banks of the world famous loch.

They arrived at the water and, having found a suitable place to pull over, they made their way to the water's edge. Gradually they plucked up the courage to dip more than a big toe into the water. A quick dip later, and a pack of howling, jabbering myths, they had all been in the water. Whether voluntarily, swimming, ducking, or being thrown in, the event was recorded on camcorder for posterity.

In Inverness the gig went smoothly, except for Charlie getting restless, getting frustrated. Maybe the burden of being driver was causing a black mood to sweep across him. Anyway, they gigged again that night then planned the next day's journey to Aberdeen.

A drive south once again, still in the North-East of Scotland, but worth their while for the views alone, Claire looked forward to the return trip to Edinburgh already.

Four hours later they were there. Fortunately Dan, the bass guitarist had brought a camcorder for the road trip, so they all amused themselves with anecdotes, silly faces, splendid views/vistas/panoramas, and other petty entertainment along the way to keep them all occupied.

By the time that they had finally arrived at Aberdeen, Claire had begun to feel a little tired, so requested a two hour kip prior to commencing the set-up for that night's gig. They located the hotel and all decided that was a good idea, so the entire band rested and grabbed a power nap. Suddenly at 7pm there was a flurry as they remembered they were on stage in two hours time, so they bolted their dinner and made for the next stop – The Grenadier's Arms.

This was a spacious pub with room for over 120 if packed out. It wasn't, though; more half full as though a group from far-removed Yorkshire were barely worth a sniff. Not that they were that bad or anything. Au contraire, Seachimp were a remarkably talented group with a fresh sound.

At 9pm they played their set, took a breather and then the second half. Over 20 discs were sold that night amongst the 80 punters milling around. The sound must have been a good one. At £10/disc, that meant £200 from CD sales in one evening. Not bad at all.

Some wise-guy requested a photo with Claire at the front of house. Charlie didn't mind; and if he did, well, it was just a photo. No need for anything rash here. Aberdeen went well all things being said.

Then it was back to the hotel, where Dan had now opened a famous Malt bottle. They spent the evening passing the bottle round, or at least, the gents did, whilst Claire went to bed earlier and supped some Apple and Melon J2O, concerned at the possible effect of alcohol on an embryo.

Charlie was getting a little stressed as he realised with a crash that he would have to be all serious and responsible for the second time in his life (on top of Fish4U!). In fact he had begun to suggest to the rest of the group that he might start a revolution and spend some of the takings on some recreational drugs. Nobody discouraged this as they were all high from the tour and inebriated from the whisky. This would have to wait, however, as there were no contacts here in the hotel.

In the morning the sun shone brilliantly through the windows. Charlie got up at 7am bright and early and decided to stretch his legs in the garden, only to find that Claire had beaten him to it. "Morning."

"Morning. What time did you get up?" Charlie asked her.
"6.30 – the sun was shining so I just got up, grabbed a fruit juice and came out here" she replied.
"Oh. Nice."
"Yeah. Busy day ahead."
"Yeah. Busy day," Charlie repeated monosyllabically.

They sat in silence for five minutes taking in the views, sounds, and atmosphere of the peaceful gardens. Claire could sense that the tour was stressing him out a little.

"Fancy some breakfast?" she asked.
"That always sounds like a plan to me," Charlie affirmed.

With that the two went inside, showered, dressed properly, then went to the dining room for breakfast.

The rest of the group congregated one by one in the breakfast hall, and they all recapped the night before. "Onwards and upwards," Claire spoke.

And onwards to Edinburgh they had determined. So that day they drove on. Here is where it happened; Edinburgh on the tour. Charlie did a bad thing that night. Once they had landed in town and located their premises to stay and to play, Charlie took himself off along with £120 of sales money. He wandered round for two hours and came back, without announcing it at first, with a pocket full of marijuana, rizlas, ecstasy tablets and a jar of poppers.

"Ok, so here's where it's at; I'll see you out front at 9pm… that's a rap", Charlie said enigmatically.

"Yeah man, you'd better believe it," said Dan unknowingly.

That night as the band played in the bar Charlie threw off his shackles and went in search of some fun. He located a likely lass and showed her a handful of tablets. "Can I interest you at all, Madame?" he inquired.

"I wouldn't go with you if you paid me," she hastily stammered.

"Fine – and I wouldn't pay you if you went with me," he retorted quickly.

By now, he was in a mood and beginning to rampage. He lit up a joint in the bar and soon attracted the attention of some interested clientele. "Hey man, have you got any going spare?" asked one guy. "I like you, I like to smoke," flirted one young lady in the bar. Charlie soon scored at twice the price with these people. At £20/eighth of an ounce he couldn't go far wrong.

Then he went a step further and began to hustle the ecstasy tablets around the clientele. "£6/pop", he began to offer. Some likely geezers came forth and bought a dozen pills for their own use later on, maybe at a club, or to sell on the streets.

From the stage Claire could see that he was getting a lot of sudden attention amongst the crowd but knew not why. Then all of a sudden she noticed a girl kissing Charlie full-on and groping him whilst attempting to dance together. Claire continued with the song at hand and felt suddenly repelled, as though a shock wave had hit her and spread right through her entire body.

By the end of the song she didn't know whether to laugh or cry, as Charlie and this other woman had vanished together out of the room. He was doing an elusive mid-tour thing, picking up strange women and abandoning all previous sense of belonging, loyalty, or other predisposed expectations.

The gig continued for the full duration, and still no sign of Charlie. There was a hubbub of activity in the bar and the band kept playing. Nobody else could have told that something was amiss, by the way they all came together and performed that night.

What were they going to do? No driver, and a set full of instruments to clear up afterwards. Where did he get to?

They finished playing by 11.30pm, and just after midnight Charlie rolled up with a head of scruffy hair, lipstick on his collar, and a look of the wild man Sam about him.

"Where have you been?" Claire demanded to know.
"Never mind, let's get cleared up for the night," he went on.

There was less talk, just a sense of angst amongst them all. She knew full well what she had seen that night.

"I saw you Charlie Morris – kissing and carousing in the front row. How could you? At a time like this? Who do you take me for?" she yelled at him.

"Oh don't be like that C, it was just a bit of fun. We're on tour for Pete's sake…"

"Yes, we are on tour – we are all on this tour Charlie, don't you forget it."

"Claire, it meant nothing, we just got carried away with the night, that's all it was," he countered.

"It meant nothing? So why did you do it, then? Because nothing is better than something after all?......what we have is something, Charlie; we have this something," patting her abdomen, "and you go off horsing round with the first thing that pulls her skirt up for you. I don't buy that."

There was an uncomfortable silence for a good long while as they packed the van and left for the hotel. Their argument had opened a whole new picture up for the band. Suddenly, they really were all in it together, and if one guy went off all of a sudden, something needed to be said.

"We've got a long drive tomorrow, back to England. Liverpool and Manchester in fact. Why not cool it for the night, big man?" Dan offered.

They did this, and cooled off for the night. That night was uncomfortable. Restless bodies in an unfamiliar place, feeling these controversial vibes all of a sudden, meant a rough night's sleep. But they got through the night and into the next morning, still alive, still surviving.

"Back to England" was the group call for the day. They had the rest of the day to sightsee in Edinburgh, so they went off in a two and a three and saw the sights, shopped a bit, and enjoyed a day of leisure.

By evening they had accumulated enough stuff for a day and then set off across the Firth of Forth and across the Borders, heading back to England.

By 8pm the van started to sputter somewhat, and by 8.30pm they were stuck in the middle of nowhere with just a mobile phone to call for help.

"Now look what you've gone and done, Charlie," Claire reprimanded him.

"Oh, do grow up, Miss Halls – we have ourselves a breakdown."

Suddenly a phone was whipped out of a pocket and a call was made to the RAC. When asked to locate themselves, that took a whole minute of map reading to figure out. "We think we've overheated," Charlie explained down the phone.

So there they were – Liverpool beckoning – stuck in the Scottish Borders on a clear night, just waiting. Waiting for action, awaiting rescue. They each took it in turn to tamper and prod about in the engine but to no avail. After 90 minutes a truck pulled up from out of the clear blue skies and the driver identified himself as the RAC man. "Let's have a look at what we've got here, then," he said matter of factly.

After 12 minutes of tapping, squirting, prodding, coaxing and tweaking, the engine was once again restarted and a thoroughly miffed Seachimp were once again reunited in their turn of fortune. "Thankyou sir, you're a star and a legend," somebody said to the RAC man.

"Ach, here's your invoice - " he replied in a Scottish accent.

They continued on their tour and arrived late that night in the city of Liverpool (European Capital City of Culture 2008). Here they simply required to do their bit the next day, get to Manchester and tour the West side of the country day by day.

Here they were in Liverpool, land of Paul McCartney, the big Macca, the big chief, the gaffer, the man that can. And Seachimp were on the bill.

Their gig went well. Charlie behaved himself and was back on CD sales. He still had some grass left over from Edinburgh, but chose to stash it in a secure left pocket rather than causing any further rift with Claire. He knew he had blundered. He would have to pay for this when they got back home again.

Seachimp played through their best tracks – 45 minutes per set. Two sets per evening with a twenty minute interval in between. There was no tell-tale sign of any argument or disturbance. The air had probably cleared since that time, just as the thunder clouds go after the storm.

They were on form. As usual, after the gig they very calmly mingled with the crowd and talked to any fans who may have come their way to ask questions. This also included meeting other stars on their way forwards in life.

Nothing gave Claire greater pleasure than to personally sign the cover of a CD in dedication to whoever was buying. That proved to her that her music was having an effect, and effect was what she wanted. Not just a pretty face singing a pretty melody, but a certain lyrical connotation at the same time.

This distracted from her disappointment in Charlie. She knew that the best person to talk to him would be Alex Davies, a mature and respected figure amongst the 'crew'. He had had years of experience and would no doubt be able to say the right things in the right way. However, this would have to wait until they returned, in 10 days time.

So Seachimp did Liverpool, then Manchester in the same light. A quick trip, and a visit around town in the touring minibus, plus much photography with their equipment. Dan's camcorder was a Panasonic; Pete, the drummer, had brought a Fujifilm digital camera with over 256MB memory available – enough for over 500 pictures to be taken.

"Bustin' loose – ain't that some funky groove", Claire announced whilst travelling. "Looks like peppercorn Charlie stole my soup," she went on metaphorically, meaning that he had upset the apple cart somewhat.

"Well, Charlie, it could be worse – death would make a mockery of us all – strike a light!" she continued.

"Ma'am, with due respect, that's in the negative trajectory," he replied with a hint of optimism in his voice.

Charlie knew full well that Claire was referring to teetering precariously on the brink as she had done not many years earlier when they first met. It would be tragic if this incident were to come between the two, now that all the happenings had been unfolding before their very eyes.

"Oh, for the elixir of youth," Claire said sarcastically.

"No need to be sarky, C – we're only human," back to Charlie.

Plan 103f

"We're on tour – time to let it go and float with the stream's flow. Thud and blunder will occur. Let's put the past behind us, moving on – Hakuna Matata," she quoted from The Lion King.

Suddenly Charlie burst into a riddle: "Throw me, throw me, but do not burn. Walk a thousand miles and pay as you earn, and with regard to reality – the door's always open but you still need a key".

"You mean like the Pearly Gates?" asked Dan.

"Simply put, dig life, not your demise," he went on with his lesson.

Food for thought as they travelled down the West Coast, on the way to Birmingham, Cardiff and Bristol. Ironically it was Charlie who was saying such things, having just gone behind her back. He was apprehensive about the forthcoming arrival. He wanted to be able to keep his 'old life' and not have to take responsibility for the unknown. The future was a scary place after all, full of uncertainty. What he wanted was a sense of certainty. That's precisely what nobody was guaranteeing.

He riddled once more, "Was it not for trials that be, transcending all along with glee, could be questioned whether would we be – living in the realms of potentiality."

"Hey man, you should take over from Jack Nicholson in Batman – the Riddler," Pete told him.

"Haa, yeah that would fit the bill," chipped in Dan.

Charlie felt momentarily blessed with these comments and continued driving with his head held a little higher because of it. Claire had an inner smile behind a solemn face. It would take more than a couple of daft riddles to win her back again.

They arrived in Birmingham and took in some sights and scenes, marvelling at the numerous 21st Century erections in town they talked amongst themselves.

"Check that out – totally phallic buildings," Claire was excited for a moment.

"Do you know to whom you are speaking?" asked Charlie, feeling put on the spot about phallic objects…"I am Torquill Van Busbo, descendant of the Grand Wazu, and when I want something doing I will not be readily dismissed," he proclaimed magnanimously all of a sudden.

"Oh, I see. And what exactly is it that you are wanting, my Lord?" She requested permission to know this detail.

"Truth is – we're so privileged. And I am grateful to be driving you people round on tour. Let's do this, let's make it a good one."

"Let's make it a good one," they all echoed.

With that in mind, the wandering ended and they focused on the gigs left yet to occur. Cardiff. Snap decision – must check out the Millennium Stadium, home of Welsh rugby, live concerts and general arena for entertainments/events. Pictures taken in and around the stadium. Seachimp had arrived.

Although they were due to perform in a smaller venue – an inn called the Merry Pipers that night – Wales was always a beautiful place to call by. The gig went well. Making a few dozen record sales and requests for t-shirts too. They were making a name for themselves now. Word of mouth had started to spread around.

People chatting on Facebook would recommend the band. Links to their 'Myspace' page were readily available, and tracks posted on 'Youtube' had thousands of hits listed by now. Seachimp were on their way up.

Then onto Bristol, making sure to call by the Exhibition Centre for a taste of the goings-on of present, they curiously wandered for a while. Bristol, then back up through the Midlands, back to Yorkshire via Lincolnshire.

"You're no monkey, Charlie" he was told.

That, in a nutshell was the Seachimp Tour round the UK, and an experience it was indeed. Everyone survived it and even the Talisker Malt came back mostly intact for later consumption.

Upon returning Claire called up Melanie, Alex's wife, and explained what had happened in Edinburgh. Arrangements were made for Alex to come and speak with Charlie. He was still not entirely forgiven despite the making-small-of-it comments made en route. She was upset still in her heart of hearts and a little confused by his sudden change of character.

There had been no expectation that he would go off selling drugs in the middle of the tour. A hidden agenda no doubt. On the face of it, this was a feather in the wind – blown by the gentlest of breezes. He had had a black mood and acted accordingly, and precious little would have affected this.

But, Seachimp were home. They had sold over 150 CD's during their tour and made a net profit of £3500. This was a start, given that some was spent on souvenirs and other memorabilia. They were back, things had happened and now it was time to make amends and get their lives back in shape once again.

Chapter 10
Charlie Morris

"Forgiveness is the fragrance the violet sheds on the heel that has just crushed it", Alex quoted some Mark Twain at Charlie. "It's not going to be easy now, you've really made a mess here," he continued. "You son-of-a-bitch, Charlie, of all the timing to go and pull a stunt like that. Have a little consideration at least, why don't you?"

There was silence for a while as both men felt angry at this time. Charlie had made a cock and balls of it, and the thought of what was just around the corner was hitting home.

"If you want to stay together now and make something, you had better pull your socks up. She would have to dig deep to let you back in, you know," Alex carried on having a go at him.

"We are all so much together but we are all dying of loneliness," quoted Charlie from Dr Albert Schweitzer. He meant that he was killing himself now he could see his errors.

They made eye contact as the gravity of the words came across.

Alex continued his lesson, "I once read some work by a Joseph Campbell, and something he said you should hear: 'It's only by going down into the abyss that we recover the treasures of life. Where you stumble, there lies your treasure. The very cave you are afraid to enter turns out to be the source of what you were looking for.' I believe you are in that abyss at the very entrance to that cave, Charlie".

"Maybe I am, maybe I'm not," he replied quietly, knowing full well that Alex had clocked his predicament to the tee.

"Don't patronise me, Charlie, I'm doing you a favour here. Remember that."

Again, an awkward silence for a moment as the two men worked through this problem. It would take more than a talking to to fully recover this situation. Claire would have to have a cool, clear and open mind to come back round to him again. They had been through a lot this last three months. There were only two months to go before the baby was born now.

"The Great, Enlightened Buddha said, 'The origin of sorrow is desire'", continued Alex.

"When the student is ready, the teacher will appear," Charlie quickly replied. Alex was doing him a favour indeed.

Meanwhile, Alex's wife Melanie was elsewhere talking through things with Claire. "We cannot change anything unless we accept it first," she quoted Carl Jung.

"My friend is not perfect – nor am I – and so we suit each other admirably," Claire responded with some Alexander Pope.

They were both getting older and wiser by the minute as they spoke together. They got onto the topic of love, and matters of the heart. "Do you love him?" Melanie asked Claire.

"Yes, I do, at least I think I do," was the reply.

"Love cures two people, the person who gives it and the person who receives it," suddenly another quote, this time from Karl Menninger for Claire.

Things began to come clearer bit by bit. She would have to forgive him and get on with life. Only, of his nine lives, he had just lost his second. That was to bear in mind. Charlie was a bit of a cat at times, and he most often fell on his feet after a fall. He now had seven lives left. How would this unfold?

To finalise their conversation, Claire asked Melanie what she could do to show her appreciation for bringing her back round to her senses. "You may not believe in God, Claire, but if the only prayer you say in your whole life is 'thank you', that would suffice"; a quote from Meister Eckhart came in handy.

So now John and Melanie had done all the talking, and it was 'job done' as far as they were concerned. All that remained was for Claire and Charlie to see what decisions they had made as a result. Both had internally decided that more important things were afoot by now so it was time to move on and put old boots to rest.

They came home independently that afternoon and Claire found Charlie relaxing in front of the television as he often would. "Hello Charles"; she used the formal name to indicate no favours.

"Hello, Claire," he replied equally formally in tone. There was no hugging or back-patting going on. After all, it had been an emotional ride for some time now. Then the ice suddenly broke and she said to him:

"Charlie, what do you call it when plan A doesn't work, plan B never occurs, and plan C isn't happening? You know what I call it? – like with you and me – to me, we are on Plan 103f – things have gone wrong; the original concept is tarnished, but we are still going, still a unit, still have things to look forward to." She tailed off with a mysterious smile on her face, flashing her teeth momentarily as though amazed at her latest concept. "You just have to keep your options open," she went on and finished with saying.

"That's the best thing I've heard all year," replied Charlie meaningfully. It was. He had heard all sorts of garbage. GIGO, he called it – Garbage-In-Garbage-Out. A common term amongst computer practitioners. He was thoroughly impressed by her. Nothing else needed to be said.

Now they had a hug, gentle and warm, minding the ever-expanding bump in her abdomen. They had experienced a breakthrough. What could have been a disaster in a tender moment had proved to be a renaissance of their original emotion. They were a team, and the rest of the crew had pulled them back together again. At least, Alex did.

What would happen next? Here's the story…both had suffered, both had united, both had been on their adventures. They now had responsibility to deal with. Would it be a boy or a girl? What would they call their child? What clothes would they buy for him/her? What food would they give? And so on and so forth. But more importantly, they had to tie the knot.

So, as she had said 'yes' some time earlier, they were already in concordance with one another. A close shave but a pull through had changed the face of it. They were going to make it down to the Registry Office within a month, in time for all parties to be informed and their own union completed.

There was no going back now, they had made their mistakes, and subsequent forgiveness and trials had proven them conclusively together. There was a long road ahead for them, and with the help of their friends they would surely make a go of things. Alex had done it again – pulling others along in times of trouble. He was used to doing so with the everyday running of the restaurant, especially during crowded periods. He was a diplomat and his assurances came in at exactly the right moment in time.

Charlie now had an eternal debt to Alex, even though Alex would hear nothing of it. Claire felt grateful to Melanie as well, for her words and wisdom. Pulling through would at least give them something to look back on, if nothing else. Life could be unpredictable at the best of times. They needed stability now and that was their new goal. They had reached an age – still young – and they wanted to settle together.

As far as material support was concerned, Charlie always believed that thoughts attract things. He was an optimist and his eye for business engaged him in opportunities on a regular basis. He was a frequent advocate of the laws of attraction. He believed that in devising specific strategies for untold amounts of money, life would present to him the means how to go about attracting that wealth into his reality.

This was not just an idea for him, or a belief – more a heartfelt conviction that he felt absolutely certain about and that would lead to an inevitable addition to his current assets. He had Claire on his side now already, and maybe life would present to him all the formulae necessary for a successful lifestyle.

Jamie Kershaw

They had met each other by the forces of attraction and had taken off on the wings of angels to a new horizon. This had never been an easy ride by any means, or by any stretch of the imagination. They had been to hell and back, and were now creating their own piece of heaven on earth. This would be their first major happiness in their lives together.

Where there was success and abundance there was bound to be an equal and opposite of some sort. After all, every action has an equal and opposite, every action causes reaction, every reaction causes consequence. Every consequence causes experience and every experience causes thoughts. Every thought causes belief, every belief causes action and so on. Charlie for one had long understood this principle and was happy to put it into action, whether it was to look for a parking place for his car, or to run the shop every day of the week. He was no fool when it came to the crunch.

The month moved pretty quickly for them and they contacted the crew one by one with an invitation. They were going to the registry office on Burniston road for the big event. Although not a huge church affair, there would be friends and family to witness the occasion. Claire had scandalised her mother by getting pregnant first, her father was just glad that they were going to hang in there together when push came to shove.

Her uncles and aunts were invited, getting on into their 60's by now. They were all proud that their niece was actually marrying her boyfriend. He was busy becoming a success in his own right. Charlie's father reluctantly accepted the invitation – he had still not fully recovered from the events of the last year or two, and his mother was happy to come.

The Registry Office would contain a bare minimum of people. Relatives present and the crew had decided to be there for this grand occasion. Just a few to witness from the crowd of 18. Alex and Melanie had come along. Ben too. He was asked to be the best man, which he had accepted, and had prepared a brief speech for the event. Shane, Suzanna, Tim and their relatives all turned up, forgetting their past differences for the time being. This was more than enough for the two of them. They were happy with this. Dressed up for the occasion in their best garb, suits and skirts – not both at the same time, mind – polished shoes and carnations in button-holes. They were a motley crew alright.

Fortunately there was no rain on the day. They went in, did their bit and then made a move to Bar2B where they had hired out the whole bar for the reception. There was a buffet and DJ to entertain everybody. Even a karaoke facility for the daring or crazy few. Claire's Uncle Steve got up to sing Lionel Richie's 'Three times a Lady', and Charlie himself got up to give a rendition of 'You're my first, my last, my everything,' by Barry White. Claire grinned wildly during his serenade.

She was glad to have a break from performing with the band. The evening went on well and people got merry and slightly drunk. Uncle Steve made a bit of a stir with his bad, loud jokes. He had the sort of sense of humour that would make the younger folk cringe. Claire could never accuse him of not trying, though.

They had a chauffeur-driven car waiting for them to take them to Bruges and Copenhagen for a week's honeymoon. They were curious about European culture, so good fortune had come their way in the form of Mr Halls snr and co who had clubbed together to pay for their once-in-a-lifetime trip. They would also take in parts of Northern France en route there and back. Meanwhile the driver was due to mind his own business and be there purely for the travelling.

They would both take it easy as the baby was due within four weeks of returning. Claire had prayed not to give birth on their travels, so Charlie began to treat her like a Queen. Now Mrs Morris, their surnames coalesced. There was a sense of permanence about the change, like a chasm of eternity gaping directly in front of her face. Was this too much?

The driver, whom we shall call Peter Houghton, was a middle-aged friend of Claire's father. An associate. Charlie would ordinarily have ditched the driver but as circumstances were so precarious it seemed right to maintain his employment. Committed to their safe transit, Peter was an expert driver and had driven on the continent more than one hundred times previously for one reason or another over the years.

He had been instructed to say little and follow orders closely. Charlie enjoyed his role as instructor very much. He had a wicked sense of humour and would sometimes get Peter to pull over to check out the sights, panoramas and vistas. Claire hardly dared move about too much. Besides, it was inconvenient.

As the tour progressed they were treated with deference by the waiters and baristas. The hoteliers ensured their comfort and privileged service whilst staying in their resort. The shop-keepers asked questions and the administration saw them to their seats for the performance - they had been given tickets to a musical in Copenhagen: Abba's 'Mamma Mia'.

They were happy and heavily weighted. Claire could have sworn that she felt kicking and jiving during the show. Charlie put his hand on the lump. There was movement alright.

At the harbour they took pictures of the famous mermaid and then retreated back to the hotel to relax in the cool of the living area. They were both anxious, so wanted to lie low for the week they were spending on the continent. Being quietly together was more than enough for the two.

They were glad to come home though, after their adventure. Back to sunny Scarborough, where all and sundry were awaiting the new arrival. They had narrowed the name list down to ten possibilities. If it was a boy then Simon, Luke, James, William, or Charles jr. And if it was a girl then Elizabeth, Joanna, Sophie, Charlotte, or Ruth would do for the Morrises. Either way, they had it all worked out by now. A new creation on the face of the earth. What if they were sick, or impaired? What if there were twins? What if Claire died during childbirth? What if a caesarean section was needed. All these doubts, and more, crossed their mind over the following weeks.

Mr Halls snr and his wife had decided to buy clothes and books already, in advance - a complete gamble given that they had no clue about the gender of the newborn. They were adamant that the Mr Men collection would suffice as first reading material for their grandchild. Ambitious as ever.

Charlie had been busy designing a spare room at home, making a play area and devising suitable décor around the room. He had an instinct for compatibility here. He would leave the painting until the following month when the baby was born.

One evening Claire suddenly felt seized by a spasm in her abdomen. "Charlie – something's happening, Charlie! Something's going on down there".

"Hold still. Remember those classes we attended. Breathe deeply, relax, be calm, think of Bruges."

"Yeah, think of fucking Bruges alright," she replied.

She sat down on the sofa and got into a comfortable position.

"Come on, let's get you out to the car," Charlie remarked.

"Yeah, let's get out to the car," she panicked.

Charlie assisted her standing up and they moved tentatively across the living room, out of the corridor and into the night air. Charlie opened the passenger door for her and she precariously entered the vehicle, swearing all the while.

Charlie got in, started the car, turned on Classic FM and began to drive to the General Hospital. They were playing a Mozart Symphony on the radio. The music served its purpose, keeping them as calm as possible during the ride.

"Oh my God, it's moving again," she yelled in exasperation.

"Moving and a grooving," said Charlie. "So long as it's alive, that's the main thing, eh, C?"

"Don't be so morbid now of all times," she retorted instantly.

They got to the hospital and Charlie, being the gentleman, rushed to get a wheelchair from the reception then came back for Claire to sit in it and be transported from the car to the building. Nurses instantly came over to make enquiries.

"She's about to give birth," proclaimed Charlie.

Quickly they wheeled her into the obstetrics department and got her lying on a bed, allowing her to change out of her clothes into something more giving. She was calling for Charlie all the time, and he was there in a flash.

"Don't worry, C, you'll be fine"

"Fine. Fuck fine! How would you know what I am right now?"

Charlie said very little at this point and held her hand tightly. He had obtained a cool, damp cloth to mop her forehead with as well. He was doing his best all the while. His greatest concern was that he was going to faint with shock at the event, but he was made of stern stuff after all.

As the night progressed Claire went into labour, contracting, screaming, and yelling obscenities at everybody. Charlie was there to utter reassurances all the while, and the midwives were hovering around waiting to do their bit.

Not until 2.30 am was the baby born. Claire uttered a final cry of the unknown and out popped a baby boy. Charlie had never experienced those giddy feelings before in his life. All of a sudden he was a father, and Claire a mother. 'Oh my, a new son,' he heard himself say. As Claire cradled the new-born he felt half proud and half envious. Claire's attentions would be elsewhere from now on.

"I like Luke," said Claire; "he looks like a Luke Morris to me," she continued.

"Wow, well, yes, indeed, Luke, that's a fine name indeed. What else was there on the list? Hmmm. Sam? David? Oh, I can't remember now. Yes, Luke Morris, that is a fine name. What about a middle name?" Charlie asked.

"Oh, that's easy.....Charles, just like his father," Claire decided in record speed. This fact had not been previously discussed. That seemed a reasonable decision to Charlie, so he concurred with a nod of the head and said, "Very well, Luke Charles Morris".

And so it stood on the birth certificate from that moment hence. A healthy baby boy weighing in at 8lb 5oz, blue eyes and the cutest tuft of hair already on his scalp. His first sound was to cry at the horror of the cold environment and bright lights. No doubt he wanted to go back into the warm, dark, liquid security he had just emerged from. This was a strange place indeed, he cried. Only, not actually saying anything as yet.

Claire held him close to her chest in her arms and jiggled him up and down. This was the biggest eye-opener of her life, bigger than winning the record contract and tour even. Charlie stood by as the early hours ticked by. Luke was placed into a crib, as both parents needed some sleep now.

They managed only four hours and by 7 am had fully woken up once again, and then the three of them had their first breakfast together in Scarborough hospital. There was an aura of a new beginning about the day as they sat together. An unbelievable challenge lay ahead of the two now, and little Luke was yet to develop a concept of the world he was born to live in. What horror, all of a sudden those distant and muffled sounds were in his face, those voices he had heard from far away were so loud and vivid. Those sensations of movement were now his own experience.

Reaching for Charlie's index finger really brought home the magnitude of his reality. Such a huge appendage for so small a hand. What else would he discover?

Besides which, Charlie took in the realm of his new responsibilities, while little Luke gazed in wonderment at the happenings of the new world he was born into. It was already a mystery unfolding at an ever increasing rate.

The three were allowed to go home together from the hospital, and so they made their way back out to the car and drove home. Charlie would have to paint the room blue or orange or green and yellow. Luke would need his own space as of now. The work would be a pleasure, an honour, a privilege. All three superlatives pretty much summed up his feelings right now.

Within 24 hours of their returning home there had been calls and visits from the relatives, gifts distributed ranging from clothes and books, to music and food items. There was no shortage of these generosities from the others.

Ben had decided to give them at least three weeks space before calling in on them again. Alex, Melanie and Fiona called in a week later to inspect the prunelike face. They were full of encouragement and willing to impart some wisdom derived from personal experience over the last five years. There was much joy and celebrating going on between them.

So what would all this mean for Charlie? He would have to love, nurture and protect his son from the outside world. Was he ready? Well, he would be as ready as he ever would be. Of that he was certain.

Two birds with one stone, the stone was Charlie Morris, the birds, well that was his business. He was an occupied man. Busy with life's offerings, and moving quickly with the times.
A 21st Century citizen, neither free from troubles nor indifferent to responsibility, he was a changed man. A reformed character. Life had shone its blessings upon him. He had asked and was now receiving.

Charlie had everything to be grateful for. He could say 'thankyou' as readily as taking a breath of air. He had come to appreciate the importance of adopting an attitude of gratitude over the years. A lot had taken place since making this transition. Once a misery in a rut, now a symbol of plenty for all the world to see. He was happy as well. Just like he hoped Luke would be in future years.

They had their work cut out for them. Claire felt more grown up now than ever before. Even more grown up than smoking cigarettes, as she once would have reasoned. They were not the point any more – cigarettes – and would only signify a downward spiral, if anything, for her. She had promised Charlie she would give up, cold turkey, and had been keeping this promise for over 10 months by this time.

He was a rock of empathy, she a font of all eternity. They were indeed a cracking good match. Mutual compassion and understanding seemed to make headway much of the time. Charlie felt obligated to conduct his business like a professional. No messing, and more to the point, looking continuously for avenues of furtherance.

Even the slightest lead could result in a significant development. Like a thread being fired from ship to ship – only, the thread was attached to a string, the string to a rope and the rope to a cable. The line connected to the other ship, and owing to the latter attachments, all the ship's crew could pass over from one to the other. Neat.

His shop ran in the same way. Nothing was ignored, nor was a call left unanswered. He had time for others, no matter how trivial it may have seemed. Sometimes a sale would be the direct consequence of his commitment here. No action would equal no result. Results were what he required.

For those days which passed like a cloud in the sky, Charlie would make efforts to hoist a mainsail and utilise the wind energy to sail his ship along. Only windless days were a concern. "No movement, what to do?" he would ask.

Wherever there was a question, the solution would present itself. At all times, in all places. That was a universal law. Ask the genie and 'Your wish is my command' he would say. 'No fear', he thought to himself. Without a shadow of a doubt there could be no accounting for changes of direction. Just as the leaves go shooting to and fro in the breeze, thoughts would fly hither and thither from the daily 50,000. It was time to get a grip, take control and establish command of his life.

Both he and Claire were very open with each other, and held no secrets. What troubled one, troubled the other. A one-time blues had become a current time ruse. They were there, a team within a team, a unit, a solid effect. There were no more obscurities between them.

As for Luke, there would be no lies told to him. They had decided to be honest all along, quite possibly fulfilling their profoundest human needs: A sense of integrity, honesty and self-respect.

Nothing could count for more at the moment. A sense of destiny shaped within themselves. Would it be good? What would unfold now? Who would come into their lives? How would they react? Why would these things happen?

More uncertainty within. Possibilities, potential for events, wholesome scope for reevaluation if needed be. Moreover, there would be room for more – people, articles, items, products, services, travels and adventures. They were unafraid of making plans, and had dreams beyond the next corner.

Plan 103f had come to them. They had worked through it and were moving on. Eventually, something had worked for them. All their previous failures had compounded, been dealt with and transformed into a learning curve and out popped a brand new solution to the problem known as the equation of life.

You didn't need to be a mathematical genius to work it out, or a rocket scientist. Sure it would help, but there was no prerogative dictating the status of any purveyor happening upon the formula. Merely, an open mind and willingness to put old problems aside and make headway with new ideas, just as the old maxim goes, 'in with the new, out with the old'.

It worked for them, it worked for everybody. Claire had a thousand reasons to be grateful for the life she had. She chose this. It seemed a valid option. Charlie had exemplified this attitude. It stemmed from Alex, too. His teachings were important enough. 'El Maestro Señor Davies' Charlie joked to him when they met.

They could afford humour between them. They were not lacking in this capacity. They were free to do what they wanted. So long as they obeyed the 'rules' of life they were free within that sphere. Charlie was a 'rules' player. He knew what constituted a good idea or materialised product, and conversely, what amounted to a worthless piece of junk.

His mind was open to this philosophical exploration. Always eyeing up the best deals, the most valuable items, or looking to invest in his future as best as possible. 'An opportunistic optimist,' just about summed him up. Others would agree.

Never one to do only a half job, or a duff activity, he tended to realise the full outcome wherever possible. He had become proud of his new role and determined to fulfil his position. Although not a school teacher, a doctor, or a lawyer, he could still convey his opinions in a coherent fashion. Still present his ideas to the world in a structured manner. Still exhibit his plans intelligibly.

Claire wanted to keep things that way at all times, for as long as was possible. She had a sense of happiness too, although was never sure what to expect.

Luke managed to play his role perfectly, an adorable, wide-eyed, bundle of innocence. All the while learning that Claire and Charlie were always present, always there, always loving, always caring, always gigantic by comparison. His own flesh and blood to look up to, at least for now anyhow. There was no reason why this should change.

Back at the 'office', Charlie went about his business like a breeze. Tasks seemed easier, chores were completed and he remained rock steady in his ways. Calls were made, thoughts always steady, emotions running through his system at a rate.

Anyhow, there would be less talk and more chalk. The Morrises were now like peas and carrots. They all went hand in hand. Chalk and cheese, birds and bees, lice and fleas, summer breeze and arctic freeze, coughs and a wheeze, pair of knobbly knees, birds and the bees, and so on.

Work was a pleasure. Even if the shop closed within a five year period he would be able to say 'We went for it, son!' and with that in mind, suddenly life seemed a whole lot brighter. You couldn't ever do better than your best. Charlie was playing full out now.

He called Claire on the phone in the afternoon. "Hello, Miss Marple, just calling to further the investigation".

"Now what investigation would that be?"

"Oh, don't you know? The mystery. The unsolved case. The file continues to grow".

"What are you talking about?"

"Don't worry, I'm just being daft. How are you? How's tricks with Lucas?"

"We're in good form, thankyou. I gave him a feed an hour ago and we've been busy playing choo-choos".

"Choo-choos?"

"Yeah. Never mind. I'll show you later".

"Can't wait".

"How's business?" she asked.

"Oh, well, steady today, but looking to pick up over the week"

"Very well. See you this evening."

They hung up their phones and continued with the day. Charlie sat at his desktop computer – a Dell – and looked on the internet, sending out emails and checking out websites along the way. This occupied him for the next two hours; he made a thorough job of it.

To his delight he discovered that there were some similar stores in Hull and Sheffield that may be willing to do business, if not impart some advice at least, ie suss out their suppliers and customer base. This was important to him, especially as the expansion was on his mind. Maybe just a backburner for now, but present nonetheless.

He had a vision to branch out when possible. This was a little ambitious though, considering the rate of trade in his current store. This was running at a foxtrot pace. Neither fast nor slow, just a steady andante walking pace. Up on two legs for sure, but not in a hurry. Charlie liked to think progressively, whether over a small or large matter; it was all important to him.

Ever ready to establish a new course when possible, he kept an eye open for the seemingly weird and wonderful. Nothing was beneath mention, or notability. The good and the bad, the black and the white, the male and the female, the yin and the yang, the hot and the cold, the solid and the liquid, the health and the sickness; all things mattered.

Fried eggs never tasted so good for breakfast. He did like a fried egg sandwich every now and again. A little bit of salt and ketchup sprinkled on top. That made his moment, especially when the yolk was still runny and made a bit of extra sauce with the ketchup. He could smile for the rest of the day after one of these.

Claire would enjoy toast, fruit, croissants, pain au chocolates, or cereal more often than a fried breakfast. Their differences didn't worry them though. They recognised their similarities, making note of what they had in common. It was too easy to follow the trends of today's society and fight everything for the cause. These two liked to focus on what was good already.

Like a leopard on the savannah merely strolling between wildebeest, lions and cheetahs. There were dangers to allow for. But best not let this rule your whole life. If Charlie had done this, nothing would ever have occurred in the first place.

A mover and shaker, a go-getter, a ground-breaking, money-making, progressive generator. Charlie could easily step out of line if it came to it, but chose to utilise the laws of gravity. If he really wanted to take off then he would simply have to design a more powerful rocket-ship engine to do the job at hand.

"I'll be your wish, your heart's desire, your rock," he told Claire prophetically one morning as they lay in bed waking up.

"Well, Charlie Morris, you go ahead and I'll be here. You know where to find me."

"Thankyou. Thankyou a thousand times. I love you".

They kissed on the lips and then one after the other they got up, showered, dressed, and went to the kitchen to make breakfast. Luke needed changing. He was making noises. Claire saw to it that that duty was dealt with. She coped valiantly.

Back to the beat. The day began, both of them feeling confident that they could meet the new challenges of the times. Charlie went ahead and made a fried egg sandwich. He put the kettle on and the bread in the toaster for Claire. They sat at the table as Luke looked on in wide-eyed wonder. They were giants. Mysterious Goliaths. Would he be David? Or would they remain a unit forevermore?

Either way he was their proudest asset. Charlie Morris was more than just a wheeler and dealer. He had become keener, meaner, leaner. Charlie Morris was a destiny-sealer and he was coming back for more.

Chapter 11
Fish4U!

Ben and Charlie would philosophise about this, that, and the other on several occasions; ranging from the price of British chips to more political agendas such as Iraq, Burma, Kenya, Zimbabwe, Tibet, the US presidential campaign, Chinese earthquakes, or Afghanistan. Whilst Ben would stand from a certain opinionated doctrine, Charlie's mind would be open to circumlocution and general transcendence from one philosophy to another.

Anyway, the point was Charlie and how he came to own his own private small business called 'Fish4U!' - how the business began to thrive, taking off the ground into the stratosphere of success.

Ever since his school days, Charlie avidly enjoyed going out to the local pub to catch a band playing a gig. He scuba-dived in the Red Sea whilst still a teenager, which subsequently inspired a passion for brightly coloured tropical fish. Only these kinds would be small enough to store in an aquarium tank, rather than big enough to swim up to a shoal of and watch them with intrigue as they suddenly changed direction.

Charlie was always an energetic boy. Slightly rebellious in his ways by birth, Charlie had energy, had focus, and a definite path to follow – that is, once he got on to opening Fish4U.

By definition, Charlie would be an independent spirit. Never one to follow the herd, or to remain in a back-seat position when in sociable surroundings; Charlie would be equally happy reading a good book alone at home, leading his business enterprise, having a raucous time on the town with the rest of the 'crew', or sitting watching a football match – supporting Middlesbrough 888.com The Reds.

Fish4U! would be his first ever real-world venture. Since he was full of courage and independent spirit, Charlie had several strategies about the direction of the shop:

1) Make a go of it:- sell fish and aquaria to people on a regular basis.
2) Make probing advances to potential clients, eg café-owners, restaurant owners such as Alex (who of course acquiesced into obtaining tropical fish for Collage, being a buddy n' all).
3) Make no probes but rely on local yellow pages to provide sufficient custom to make a living.
4) Make an application to the lottery fund for an extension and to turn the shop into a more general pet shop.
5) Cut and run (no real intention here).
6) Go bust, drop the dead donkey and sit in the local pub wheezing his life away.

As the only options to appeal to Charlie would be to make a go of Fish4U! he opted for strategies #1 and #2…making tactful visits to all sorts of local cafés, coffee shops, bistros and restaurants with the real intention of selling some tropical fish. And guess what? He got the custom that kept him afloat. Although most Scarborians would have preferred to eat the fish with their chips, he found to his delight that some were willing to pay a pretty penny to amuse themselves for hours gawping at beautiful fish swimming about the tank.

"A thousand miles in a thousand days have I travelled and there is nothing I would rather own than my own tropical fish for my living room" said one old customer.

"God bless ya," replied Charlie as he helped him choose his fish. "Only remember – no cats sir – not if you value your fish, now".

Good times for all like this were regular occurrences for Charlie as Fish4U! attracted many an interesting individual. There would be no fun having these bright fish if the fish had no names. So when not prospecting for custom, Charlie would feed the fish and call them names like Zippy, George, Alan, Florentine, Albert, Mona, Betty, Sue, Simon, Dave or John. He had a lot of fun naming his fish like this.

Charlie's way was with style. A real flair for making things work out just fine. Charlie's way involved trial and error. He would happily make mistakes on his journey forwards. In fact, to not make some sort of error would be anathema to his learning etiquette.

So, moving on, with the tropical fish 'n' all, we could see Charlie simultaneously running a business and a relationship with Claire. From time to time she would run errands for him as well, helping with a delivery to a customer, or running back and forth in the van to the suppliers with some new fish. They both loved to visit the Sea Life Centre on a weekend when all was quiet. They enjoyed watching as the assistant would feed the seals and the penguins. They loved to see the fish swimming round, the sharks, the seahorses and anemones. It seemed to add an education to their list of what-to-do's.

Charlie had been inspired by Alex through and through. The fact of setting up one's own small business and making a go of it really appealed to him. So, lo and behold, Fish4U! was born. Although his daylight hours would be entirely consumed with business dealings, the fish shop provided a place of karmic repose for him. He felt good about it. He had a sense of responsibility, a sense of determined effort and a feeling of valuable social contribution which could not be denied him now. Charlie was no genius, nor a budding musician or athlete, but he sure had the balls to start up a business enterprise of his own accord.

Maybe they were natural, maybe they came about only from being with Claire, maybe they came from following his dream, his heart and prerogative. Whatever difference it made, Charlie was able to set up his business and make a go of it.

"Babe, we've got a big haul coming tomorrow".
"OK, just give me the address, and I don't mind going at all".
"Well, it's not just that, you see, there's a direct payment to be made as well."
"Oh, I thought they had covered that already?"
"No, not yet. They came out with a million reasons why they would only pay on delivery…"
"Suchas?"
"…oh, I don't know. I don't want to go into all that now, anyhow".
"Ok, fair enough. I'll see what I can do."
"Thanks C, you are a star!"

"I know."

With that they continued on the day's work in the shop. Charlie began talking to the fish in the tank and fed them some dry flakes.

"You're so considerate, you know."
"You betcha. These little beauties deserve the best, now hear".
"Haaa haaa. You've got a funny way with words, you know."
"Yes, I'm a positive thesaurus when I want to be".
"OK then, tell me, Mr know-it-all, how would you talk of your enterprise in other words?"
"Oh, that's easy enough C. Ask me another will you? For starters there is venture, trade, project, operation, proceeding, endeavour, initiative, dealings and so many more".
"Oooh, now I'm impressed"
"Good, I'm glad. Nothing more to say now. Back to it!"

With that, the two got on once again in the shop. Claire began to contemplate her next gig lined up that night. She was dying to do some solo stuff as well as appear with the band. Seachimp were beginning to get on her tits by now. All the rehearsing time was a little bit chaotic to say the least. The band consisted of Claire on acoustic guitar (when solo) or electric guitar and lead vocals, a bass guitarist, drummer, keyboard and a flautist/mouth organ player. So, a simple set-up in all.

Thinking to herself she thought 'sometimes the simplest things in life are the most beautiful', 'if music be the food of love, then Guinness be the food of life', 'too many thoughts for my poor simple head now', 'only, what if it transpires that I am more complex?', 'wouldn't that be funny?', 'yeah I like the sound of that', 'Complicated lead singer takes Seachimp to a whole new level!'

"Hey Charlie…do you think I'm too complicated?"
"A positive Galileo, dear"
"Seriously, I mean"
"Why do you ask all of a sudden?"
"I was just thinking"
"Oh right, thinking out loud. Fair enough"
"Well, my music is simple, but we're all complex people".

"Most important"

"Don't be sarcastic with me, Charlie"

"Heaven forbid"

"Why are you being so rude?"

"C, I think your music sounds great. You and the rest of Seachimp have a lot of potential to go all the way. Truly."

"You do mean that, don't you, Charlie?"

"Yes Claire, yes I do. I love your stuff and you know I do."

"Yes I do know that."

"But you must remember – Outside the art an artist must never dream."

"That just says it, Charlie – you're right"

The two collaborated for quite some time before they got on once again. The day's work was lined up and they hustled and bustled and mulled over thoughts, turned over the accounts book, kept the shop clean and tidy, spick and span, up and running, and she got onto thinking about the gig that night.

"Maybe they will like our new tracks? I hope so – they better had now with Mark on the ol' tin sandwich".

"Don't worry C, chill out and relax while you can. If you want to get off a bit earlier that's a-ok with me. There's not much doing today and I don't mind closing shop if you need the time"

"Yeah, but what if we make a cock-n-balls of it? That would kill the whole show".

She proceeded to lay it on thick, a whole panoply of melodrama and thoughts of detriment until they had reached an agreement.

"There are to be no cock-n-balls here in the shop. We are an up and running enterprise with no room for that kind of eventuality. So you run along home now and rest your bones and leave me here in charge of the store. I will see to it that the day's tasks are accomplished" Charlie affirmed.

"Oh, very well then, you're the boss. I will do then. So back for tea?"

"Yes Mrs, I will be back for tea – you go and see to the child and I will see you later."

Charlie sent her on the way and began to clear up the shop front with a broom. There was a bit of rubbish lying around on the ground. He also got a cloth and bucket of warm, soapy water and proceeded to clean the shop window. Not that it needed a clean, but more to keep occupied and to look busy to any passers-by looking on.

It was 3pm by now and another two hours to go in the shop. Would there be any more orders coming in for the day? Or would it be a quiet one? He had the potential to earn over £250/day when sales were going well, or over £1000/week when the going was good. Some days he would receive orders up to his ears, whereas other days like today, were on a relative stand-still.

Standing on tip-toes he reached high for a shelf with some empty cardboard boxes on them. He figured that they could be useful for storing some old files in. So he went to work and arranged the unwanted, unused files and then placed them in order into the boxes. That is, by month and year. With one month per file there were at least 15 to sort out.

He liked to regulate the administration like this, in order to keep on top of the matter. That day there were no more orders but he was curious to find out how his son was getting on. Any wailing or puking to be reported would soon be uncovered by the call home.

He returned home to a very quiet household. Claire was resting on the settee and Luke was having a sleep in his cot. What was apparent to Charlie was that she would have to prepare for tonight's gig leaving him in charge of the baby. Whatever was he to do? He had been in less compromising positions before but the classes he had attended had taught him how to change a nappy and console a wailing infant.

Poo smells, stains, wet patches, sick down the shirt front all had to be allowed for. And what's more, Luke could get mighty raucous if he wanted to. Especially when hungry, he would yowl out loud.

Claire had understandably taken a breather; "You go Charlie – your turn".

"I've only just got in," he would say in return.

"Yes, well, I've been at it all afternoon and now you can go and be a good father," she suggested succinctly.

"Oh, bugger it, alright." He went over to the cot and picked up Luke in his arms, gently rocking him up and down as he cried for a while. He needed a change, so Charlie did the deed in seconds flat. He had become experienced in the matter by now.

Luke soon calmed down again so he was given a dummy to chew for a moment until it was spat out along with a mouth full of drool. 'Splendid,' Charlie thought to himself.

"And just think, no money in all the world could have bought me my baby Luke," he told Claire as she rested still.

"Yes, just think, indeed," she replied non-commitally.

"You know, the best part of it is that he always calms down again afterwards. A bit of warm milk and a mashed up Farley's Rusk and Bob's your Uncle," he explained to her.

"There's more to it than that, to be sure," she said in an Irish accent for some reason. "Anyway I had better get ready for the gig tonight now, had I not?"

"And just leave me here all that time?"

"I'll come back, you'll see," she promised.

All that mewl and puke seemed to have a point, and for Claire and Charlie it was a lesson in growing up. A steep learning curve at that, and one full of challenges and other experiences to accompany. "Join the club," she said.

Claire woke up fully and began to think about the night's gig. Charlie would stay in and be a responsible dad. Luke would stay in and be a blessing to the world. Together they would pull together and be a unit. The crew were proud of this. People thought highly of Charlie and had been impressed with how far he had come on since his ASBO some time previously. Claire felt that he was to be trusted with her infant. He would take care of him in a decent manner.

Seachimp were due to play in town again, and had – by now – picked up some major credentials amongst their regulars. Their reputation had grown following the tour promotion. Word had spread around, to be sure. They were beginning to take off in a big way. Claire was relieved to have had a successful birth and to have been able to continue singing and playing as well. If it wasn't for the music, she would never have met Charlie in the first place.

Charlie felt riveted in an anxious way about the evening's responsibility. He would have to play the role which he had been prepared to play for a long time. Simultaneously going through joy, happiness and good spirits – known to the Greeks as Eudemonia – he also felt apprehensive about his role. Would Luke be too much to deal with?

Her last words to him that evening before going out to the gig were, "Be strong dear – firm but fair". She waltzed out of the door and headed to meet the rest of the band, leaving Charlie to do his job at home. There was to be no rest for the wicked tonight.

Luke remained calm most of the time, so Charlie picked him up and rocked him gently in his arms, intrigued by the gurgles and splutters, grins and mirthful sounds coming from his son. "Dada," it sounded like at least. Was he just imagining these to be his first words?

Walking up and down the living room there was the sound of Yorkshire Coast Radio on in the background at a soft volume. They were playing a selection of lively tunes throughout the session interspersed with DJ commentary, news updates and people ringing in to express their views.

Claire would be back home by 11.30pm at the latest, so there was nothing to worry about. The evening was fairly eventless all in all.

No real wailing or vomit or messed pants or anything. When she got in, Charlie was in the living room drinking a hot cup of Horlicks.

"Whaddup, Charlie Brown?"
"Watcha"
"Is he sleeping?"
"Yes, he's been quiet for a while now"

She disappeared into the bedroom to make an inspection and returned a minute later.

"Yes, he looks so cute – so tiny and cuddly – when he's asleep," she went on.
"Good gig?"
"Not bad at all, in fact – no hecklers. We played two sets tonight in all. Seemed to go down a treat."
"A treat, huh? Can't be bad"

They sat for a moment and then had a cuddle for a moment. It would be back to work tomorrow in the shop on a Thursday. Who knows, maybe there would be some orders coming in?

They went to bed soon after, switched off the lights and got some sleep. Only they were woken three times in the wee small hours by Luke's complaints. He cried in the night and needed an early morning feed. This was Claire's department.

In the morning the alarm went at 7.30am. Charlie got up first and took a shower. He came back into the bedroom and proceeded to get dressed. He gave Claire a gentle shake on her right shoulder. "Coffee?"

Big yawn and an arm stretch then a cross between a coherent response and an indifferent rolling over on her other side. Charlie said "I'll take that as a 'yes' then, chick."

He went through into the kitchen and made a bit of breakfast – toast and a banana. He then took a cup of white coffee through to Claire in the bedroom. "Here, this'll wake you up" he mentioned. Then he went through to inspect Luke "You'll be coming with us today fella," he told him.

He meant business. Today he was going to show Luke the shop from an inside perspective, from the point of view of the shop-keeper. In this case, Charlie. Fish4U! was a thriving enterprise these days. There was custom, there were customers, there was a constant turn of events ensuring that things could unfold within. There were jobs to do and work to be done.

'Never a dull moment here,' thought Charlie. He worked hard and played hard, believing that 'all work and no play makes Jack a very dull boy'. He followed a healthy survival credo every day, involving integrity, diversity and determination. He did like to diversify where possible. This meant that he could experience a voyage of discovery as new ideas cropped up and schemes developed. He did not wish to let things fall stagnant if at all possible.

Sometimes things just had to count. There came times when the hours and hours of hard work began to pay off. Occasionally it could be merely seconds that counted. A telesale, for example, or a face-to-face encounter where presentation meant everything. A lot could be said for those first moments of encounter.

Claire finished her breakfast and then they all three went together (Luke strapped onto Charlie's back) to the store and opened up for the day ahead. It was a new day indeed and there was much to be accomplished therein.

They had an agenda to keep to, so determined to keep to it. With digits, figures, fish to feed, tanks to keep clean, calls to make, prospective clients to impress and otherwise maintain a thriving business they had their work cut out for them for the day. Luke's demands kept them equally on their toes, moment by moment. He would point at the fish and squeal triumphantly as they swam towards his finger on the glass tankside. He looked in awe as they swam to the surface to eat the dried fishflakes that were sprinkled there. Many colours were represented amongst the miniature shoals within the tanks. There were stripes, dots, plains, short, fat, long, and thin.

Charlie had planned to make some sales that day. With this in mind he sat at the desk and picked up the telephone. One call lead to the next, to the next, to the next - restaurants, hotels, bars, and other pet-related stores in the area and further afield in the county.

With all this hard work and abundance of cold-calling he made precisely no sales today whatsoever. A waste of effort? Never a waste as far as Charlie could see. 'Nothing ventured, nothing gained,' was his motto.

He sat for a moment and blew out a huff of air, a forceful breath in consolation at his nul-points scoresheet for the day. There was plenty of time, and so the remainder of the day was turned into a maintenance occurrence. He made things ship-shape and even contacted the local gazette to make a month's marketing ploy within the daily circulation.

The truth being told, this was his best bet within the local community. Although he had his eyes on a bigger picture as well, looking to expand more nationally to the South of the country and the northern extremities too.

Meanwhile, Claire and Luke were out on a walk in the sunshine. Taking in the views and vistas along the way, they enjoyed their jaunt on this day very much. Stopping for a sandwich in a café near the beach and a refreshment as well they spent two hours away from the shop today. Charlie was glad to see them back again once they had made up their minds to return.

The day was not as productive as they may have liked. Plenty of calls and forwards moves but no darned sales whatsoever. The question they were asking was, if this continued how long would they thrive for? Would the business collapse after all? How could they pull back up into the stratosphere once again?

As yet this day would just be a flash in the pan, a slow day of nil effect. It couldn't go on like this, anyhow. There had to be a way back into the profitable environment. Whether by hook or by crook he would find a way to make those sales. He had to, the shop relied on this.

They were family now, Claire, Charlie and Luke. They had been through a rough patch and a sense of detriment, but this had all been surpassed by now, probably owing to the guidance of Alex their friend. Had he not put in a word when he did, there would be no telling of the outcome in the meantime.

Anyhow, Fish4U! was still going and there were gigs coming in from various angles. They had learnt the value of team-play over the last two years, and now it was being tested with both thrown in at the deep end of the pool. Charlie was used to challenges; throughout his life he had known challenges.

He was glad that they had managed to pull through and carry on regardless. He did realise that he had behaved irresponsibly and felt honoured in a way that it had all worked out like this. He had his enterprise, his business baby, and now he had his biological baby as well. More than a handful, to be sure.

Charlie was intrigued every minute of every day and was keen to play the part. Even though they had made no sales on this one day, he would not let it get him down. It was all part and parcel of running a small business, he told himself. Anyhow, there were other considerations these days, too.

He had called Ben in the afternoon to see if he wanted a tank for his office at work. Ben had other priorities on his agenda. "Oh, hi Ben – Charlie here"

"Hello, Charlie, what can I do for you?"
"Well, actually, I am calling to sell you an aquarium complete with fish."
"Ohhhh, so you're having a slow day then, I take it?"
"That's not the point – well, yeah actually, kinda slow."
"Hmmm, well, I have to say 'no can do' I'm afraid. My hands are tied with Pépé right now and he's more than a handful"
"Oh, right, well I thought I would try"
"Yes, no harm done now; oh, regards to your others, by the way"
"Thanks Ben – will do."

And the call ended. A 'friendly' as it turned out. There was never any telling how it would unfold with it being a sales call and all. He had to take his hat off to people for being so diplomatic about it, even though they were rejecting him. But it always made a splendid change to hear the words, "I'm interested, actually; hold the line while I write some stuff down".

Moments like these were breakthroughs and not to be ignored. Anyhow, today was a 'slow' day so he decided to wind down earlier and take a walk to the park with Claire and Luke. They enjoyed the sunshine and took in the views. People seemed to treat them a bit differently now they had Luke. Even like royalty in some cases.

Charlie needed to develop a new strategy, so he asked Claire what she thought about the matter. "What do you think, Claire?"

"Well, we live in an ever-changing world of constant fluctuations, tides, winds and energy matter"

"Yes, I like it" said Charlie. He went on, "So how come there are no sales, then?"

"That is part of the seasonal cycle. It takes a new start-up to react with interest," she suggested.

"But, I really need a strategy, not just philosophy."

"Hmmm, you know your basic four – product, price, promotion, place – "

"Fish4U!, £185, tropical fish, Scarborough - North Yorkshire"

"Well there you go, then. You've got your basics, just expand on this a little."

"Ok, clever clogs, here's a deal then – we up the prices, contact 8 more counties with related businesses, and incorporate more equipment as well."

"Genius idea, bound to work, you'll see," she winked.

Charlie took pride at his flourish of an action plan. Now he had an idea what to do, he just needed to put it into action. So they walked on and chuckled to themselves at some inane jokes they made. The afternoon was very pleasant and nothing wasted.

The next day when he opened shop he went straight for the web and located stores in East, West, and South Yorkshire. He made at least 25 calls by lunchtime and already things were beginning to pick up somewhat. Three of the stores had expressed an interest and had offered to send a representative to visit personally and make an inspection for potential clientele.

Charlie hadn't said 'no' to that, so he was in good spirits when he saw Claire at lunchtime.

"So your foolproof plan is working then, Charlie Brown?" she asked nonchalantly.

"No-one said it was foolproof," he uttered, "but yeah, there is some interest out there. Somebody, somewhere loves me, baby!"

"I wouldn't count on it if I were you," she remarked back.

He grinned from ear to ear as Luke crawled around the carpet curiously. It was like seeing life that mattered. Claire scuttled across to pick him up again. "He keeps getting his hands all dirty," she told Charlie, "the daft sausage."

Charlie went through to the kitchen to make a sandwich and munched it fervently. He had settled for a ham salad today with a glass of lemonade. "Ain't ever seen such a sight as you," he said to Claire.

"What's that supposed to mean?" she retorted

"Nothing, just that you're the best."

She looked at him with raised eyebrows for a moment then devoted more attention to Luke.

"I'm going back now," he said, "so see you later."

He returned to the shop and made some more calls from the desk. There were a couple of messages left on the answer phone as well to deal with. He decided that the new price for a tank of 12 fish should be £225 with a 12 month guarantee. He knew that the fish may not live much longer than 24 or 36 months, so didn't want his customers coming back all the time with dead fish to renew.

Also, he had his eyes on entering a partnership with a 'brother' organisation when he could find any interest. Would that day come? Maybe, maybe not; he would have to wait and see. Fortunately he was a patient chap and this was something he could bank on doing – that is, waiting patiently.

The rest of the day was spent taking specific actions to further the store and its name. He had previously ordered 1,000 business cards to distribute around the area. He was going to deliver them by hand, to as many addresses as possible, maybe even with some photographs of the fish so that people could see he meant business. The cards hadn't arrived yet, so that was to be waited on for another day. Basically, he had his work cut out for him. Designing a web page would never be easy, but that was another idea to elaborate on.

He really desired a trip to return to the Red Sea to see the fish up close again as a scuba diver. He had been there before as a young teenager, and had thus been inspired all along. Or the Indian Ocean, Great Barrier Reef, Florida Keys, or somewhere as good would do equally well, he had decided.

As for place, he was chuffed to even have a location in the first place, but his eye was always on that next step. What can I do to improve on this little bit here, or there? Where can I go next to make that all-important connection? How should I get there? Who with? Why do I even want to do this in the first place? All these questions and so many more featured as principally important for Charlie now.

He had an intelligent mind. He was blessed to have a thought process that made sense to himself and to others. He wasn't the only dog in the neighbourhood either. On speaking with Alex, Charlie had come to terms with his own shortcomings and been able to reevaluate his misguided notions. In short, he was on the straight and narrow, and it was down to Alex that he had decided to see it through with Claire and Luke.

That was established by now, and things were making sense. At least, that is the stance that seemed to be accepted already. As for Ben, well, he was only too happy to communicate with Charlie as well. Whether about a business consultation, a philosophic discourse, or a mere friendly chat, Ben could be relied upon by Mr Morris. He was now known as 'The Professor', amongst the crew.

Charlie was glad for him that things had been evolving in his own life. It wasn't all sitting in his ivory tower. Some days there were bells and whistles to show for it. These were the days which Ben looked forward to. The days when something could be seen, or some profundity enunciated. He liked to show off from time to time. There were no better people to show off for than Claire and Charlie.

They were his best and fondest audience. He did have his points to make, and his contributions for the shop were often valid and welcomed. Ben had his own work cut out for him as well up at the campus. The students were not getting any easier, or younger. He was able to teach, entertain, enlighten and instruct all at the same time. For Charlie, he was invaluable.

Fish4U! was very much up and running. There was more than one person on board this freight train. Charlie had input from many different sources, a business plan in action, some new strategies to develop, a fully operational scheme, and he had interest more to the point. 'Where there was a will there was a way,' he thought often.

His secrets were secrets only amongst the chosen few. He had plans and in order to make them work he had been talking to the crew. In talking to the crew his dream had come into fruition. He owned his tropical fish shop, he had Claire, they had Luke. Life had been transcending the usual routine recently - where Charlie Morris walked, people were bound to talk. "Fish4U!, sir? Fish4U!, madam? Just call, we'll deliver to your door."

Chapter 12
Tim's Struggle

Tim would get up early in the morning to train before going to work at J Sainsburys. Being ambitious he would often rise at 5am and train for two hours, normally in the swimming pool, before stretching off, cooling down and preparing for a day's work ahead to pay the bills. He lived in a small apartment near the town centre of Scarborough, but so long as there was room for his bike that was all that mattered to Tim.

It had been going on for months before there were any signs of strain on him. It had seeped in bit by bit, not at all quickly, but more of a subtle inner tension building up little by little until it had reached a level at which Tim would feel 'stressed out'. He figured that this was part and parcel of his athletic ambitions, so just carried right on with the early mornings, full days and home by six o'clock in the evenings. Three days a week he would train in the evenings as well, either cycling or running. The swimming sessions were always reserved for the early mornings before other people woke up and arrived for their own swim.

The London Team GB trials would be fast approaching now that the summertime loomed ahead. These results would determine his fate. Would he be good enough for the Olympic Games? There were no indications to say he wouldn't be at least a top ten finisher, although he distinctly had hopes set on winning the race, as ever. Given his commitment to the triathlon over the last three years his goal would often be realised in smaller meets. His coaches knew he stood a good chance.

Sponsors perked up steadily since he won the Ripon, North Yorkshire Triathlon in 2008. Asics and Reebok decided to forwards some kit to him. Training shoes, socks, shorts, underwear, t-shirts and also some Speedo swimwear. Much to his delight he was beginning to receive favourable attention. The local gazette wrote of his achievements in the sport section every fortnight.

Tim had the added advantage of support from the Jeffries' siblings Shane and Suzanna. Also triathletes, these two were never in the same league, but sure as sure they would train together in the mornings sometimes and cycle in the evenings.

Shane and Suzanna were on the county squad for men and women respectively, but did not have the extra ounce to make the national teams. They were, simply put, overshadowed by faster athletes. Both extraordinarily fit in their own right but beaten to the mark when it came to the crunch. Tim had proved himself to them on countless occasions and needed no further explanation. Both were secretly hoping that he would be selected for the Team. Maybe envious at the same time, but out of competitive rivalry they knew he had a very real chance, and would be happy to see someone they knew flying high and dry at the Olympics.

So the three would train together and meet up on a regular basis. But the killer came one evening in November time.

Tim woke up in the middle of the night with a bad head. Suddenly, out of the darkness of night, everything came crashing home. He would never win Olympic Gold. The deluded young fool.

Thinking to himself: "I don't understand. Why am I suffering now of all times? Questions, questions, all these questions. I'm on my own, I know that much. Nobody is going to send me there on a silver platter. Lord, I'm really going to have to work hard for this."

"What was it the guru said about good fortune? Yeah, Tony Robbin's wisdom 'when preparation meets with opportunity, this generates the offspring that we call luck'."

"I am ready though, after all that training. I know grandpa Billy ran a marathon at the 1960 Rome Olympics. He didn't win but sure as sunshine he was there on that course. My folks have no real faith in me. The bible says 'For all their seeing they may not see, and for all their hearing they may not understand' (Luke 8:10)."

He reasoned that a true friend would stand by him no matter what, then managed another rough two hours sleep before getting up again at 5am to go for a swim. Suzanna had agreed to meet him at the pool for training that morning.

Tim met her at the door and explained his rough night to her. They began to talk more optimistically.

"We live in a world of paradigms" said Tim.

"How do you mean?" asked Suzanna.

"Everybody is different. Unique."

"Go on, explain…"

"I'm a sports person. You are too. Benjy is an academic. Alex and Charlie run businesses. Claire is a musician. So on and so forth."

"Well, thanks for stating the obvious, Mr Wise Guy", retorted Suzanna.

Tim carried on "I'm not done yet. The paradigms of the living. You know, a scientist lives for experiment. An artist lives for creation. A chef lives for recipes. A businessman lives for capital. We all have a specific purpose, a destiny, and these paradigms define our boundaries."

"Define a paradigm."

"Alright" said Tim "….a set of rules or assumptions about what people can or cannot do towards achieving their goals."

"Ohhhh, right. So a creative musician, like Claire, would not get too far studying the structure of some modern architecture?"

"No, but she would still stand to learn something from this, either way."

"Yeah, isn't that just great. Ain't it great mate, haaaaa."

The two had a good laugh, then entered the building.

Tim went on: "A game of tennis is a perfect example for a life paradigm...one person delivers the problem to the other and each player takes a turn to solve their problem and provide an alternative problem back again. The winner is the one who can cause the other to be unable to solve their problem."

"You're getting complex on me now" said Suzy.

"Imagination is more powerful than the intellect."

"So said Einstein. Even I know that much."

"You know what the essence of each new day is for me? When I wake up in the morning I remind myself that whatever you can do or dream you can, begin it. Boldness has genius, magic and power within it. Goethe said that."

"You are a wise boy, you know that?"

With that they commenced their training session in the pool. Suzanna was thinking about what was said and after the session at 7am they began talking once again after changing.

Suzanna "One of my favourite quotations...without the heart there can be no understanding between the hand and mind...Madonna."

In jocular mood "Ok, yeah I like it. Le Maillot Jaune.....everybody wants it and when you've got it, nobody else can have it."

Continuing, he said "Yeah; paradigms. It's all good."

"You could *be* that opportunist Tim. You know...carpe diem and all that? The question is, when do you stop? When do you know how to stop?"

"Until she shines baby, until she shines - a playful wind knows how to stop at will."

Suzanna reflected: "I remember an inspiring passage I read in the bible: 'But they that wait upon the Lord shall renew their strength;

they shall mount up with wings as eagles; they shall run and not be weary, and they shall walk and not faint' (Isaiah 40:29-31)."

After their session the two athletes went their separate ways until the next meeting.

Tim had pushed himself hard that morning during the swimming session, and then spent a half hour doing yoga and breathing exercises. No change there from his usual routine. He had gone to Sainsburys for the day's work as ever and found it fairly standard as far as a working day in a supermarket ever went. However, that evening, he met Shane and decided that they would ride a forest trail which had been on his mind for quite some time by now.

Shane knew the route as he had studied it on a map previously. So both youths set off on their bikes. Suzanna wanted to relax that time instead, so stayed at home. They set off with their bikes and made their way towards Dalby forest some fifteen kilometres down the road. As the ride was to be forty kilometres, that gave them at least ten kilometres on the forest trail.

They took a mobile phone, two water bottles full of lucozade sport, and wore crash helmets – their two fighting-fit bodies racing along on a warm spring evening.

As they arrived in the region of the forest they noticed a dozen other cyclists preparing to ride as well. They knew their route, however, so carried on at a rate of knots.

Down hills, and racing along narrow, rocky paths with tree roots sticking out at peculiar angles along the way. Both cyclists confident that the ride would provide some extreme fun for them. Tim took off over the roots, Shane followed close behind. They picked up pace and suddenly there was a fallen tree right across the path. Tim hit it full on. He jack-knifed straight over the top of it and landed in a heap on some solid ground. Shane followed suit within a split second.

"Aaaaaargh!"
"Whooooooah!"
"…where the hell did that come from?"

"Are you hurt?"
"My arm's tingling a bit"
"Fuck - I think it might be broken"
"No way. You alright?"
"Yeah, just some bruises and grazed knees"
"Let me see your arm. Can you move your wrist?"

Tim spent a moment of consternation as he tried to rotate his wrist.

"Damn - that hurts!"
"Man, I think its broken. I'm going to phone Suzanna"

Shane reached in his bike bag for his mobile phone and made the call.

"Suze, it's me…"
"…we had an accident in the forest. Tim broke his arm…."
"…no, not cyclists. A log across the path. We smacked right into it on the way. Can you drive to the forest to pick us up with our bikes? Tim needs to see a doctor."

"That's great. See you in twenty minutes by the reception cabin. Thanks Suze, you're a lifesaver"

And with that the call ended and Tim's worst fears began to come out to the forefront. "What about the trials, Shane? I'm damned if I miss them with a broken arm. These mean the world to me. After all that training, and now this. I'm not going to miss those trials in May no matter what happens. I can still run!"

"They wouldn't let you if you had a cast on. Give it time and see how you heal, dude."

Both knew this could be bad news for the next year's trials.

Twenty minutes later Suzanna arrived; the two boys had pushed their bikes back down to base on foot. Silently, in pain, running through his potential exclusion in his mind Tim knew out of instinct that that log would cost him his place unless he could heal quickly.

******

The doctor gave him an instant x-ray when they arrived at the hospital the next morning. There was indeed a fracture of his left wrist. And with that, Tim found himself ushered into the next room for a cast to be set on his arm. He worried now. Now that he would have to be wearing an addition to his usual appendage, he was concerned about recovery, keeping fit (known as maintenance), and more to the point, about his trials forthcoming in May. He would not be able to attend if it were anything to do with a fractured wrist and a plaster cast.

As he emerged from the surgery in a state of abject misery Suzanna greeted him with the words, "That's a cracker – get it?!"

Tim was not amused. He merely snarled and bared his teeth at the prospect. In fact, he had begun to formulate a plan of action already. He was going to take Ben up on his mentoring offer. You know, to tread the water and see what bright ideas would emerge from him now he was in this predicament.

After all, the cast would remain only three weeks maximum, and Tim would still be able to walk and jog with relative ease. Cycling and swimming would prove to be more of a problem for him in the immediate term.

As it happened, Ben had an instant solution for Tim – a quick fix, in fact. You see, Ben was the proud owner of an electronic exercise bike at home, and he had no feelings of purely self-centred ownership as to keep it all to himself. As soon as the situation had become apparent to him, he made a pact with Tim – "come over to my place three times a week to cycle on the machine".

"Yeah – consider that a done deal, my good man."

"The deal is delivered with a seal, dude – if I may? – I have a training programme in mind to get you to your trials in May regardless of your arm. The seal is: You use my bike, and I'm still your mentor."

"Well, I would need to be persuaded more advertently, you see. But there is less time to refuse this most generous offer than would be plausible. It does seem rather that I will have to take you up on your offer of a bike-mentor deal. Crikey, what a facility after all!"

"My name is Benjamin Williams and I profess only to the best!"

"Don't start up on your trumpet now, Prof. I will be there on Tuesday morning – name a time, or cut me a spare key. They will give me time off work at Sainsbury's now. To be honest, I could do with the extra time to rehabilitate."

The two gentlemen conversed for a while longer and then they signed off. Tim already began to feel more confident that he could keep on track for the trials next year. He turned back to Suzanna and said:

"Miss Stevens, it would seem that we are onto a winner after all!"

"Jolly good, boyo. Maybe we can get some lunch. Fancy a trip to the café?"

"That would be cool. We get to show off this monstrosity to Alex and Melanie," (referring to his plaster cast). "And that's only the beginning. Anyway, when is your next shift?"

"Tomorrow morning setting up for lunch, and staying all day for the evening scene, too."

"OK. That's cool".

Whether it really was cool or not is another question, but the two were kind of warming to each other in a non-triathlon fashion. Maybe there would be something extra lurking behind the doors of external perception. Who knows, maybe these two would stick it out through thick and thin and thus form an utterly inseparable bond as surely as the Power Rangers roamed.

Would Ben be a hindrance? Would he be invaluable? Maybe there would be nothing more than a platonic relationship between them all. What did Suzanna intend? What else was on Tim's mind? Anything else? Or was he 110% focused?

All these questions to consider and turn over. The facts.... Tim burned and yearned for the Olympic Games; Suzanna remained loyal with local café culture, Ben had a new position to fulfil responsibly. Surely there would be no time for a love triangle?

'What chaos that would be,' Suzanna thought to herself as the thought emerged in her mind. Literally so, as it would seem; just as a field of bullocks smacks of testicles, so would a love triangle.

Perhaps she simply wasn't ready to strike up an intimate relationship. The crystal-clear goals were there within Collage and The Flaming Squirrels. The values all made perfect sense as well, which was a bonus. The working ethic where everybody would know where exactly they stand, what to do and how much time there would be to do it in. Suzanna knew that she could keep on training with a little guidance.

Tim was bugged out, man. He was now down to a morning session consisting of yoga and deep breathing, and four days he would walk to Ben's place to use the exercise bike for 20km at a time. He read Cycler's Weekly and Runner's world and Triathlon 220 magazines to get inside inspirations. He gained a lot of significant knowledge from reading these publications.

Anyway, now that his arm was broken and in a sling, he had to concentrate more on what Ben was saying. Shane was a constant buddy to Tim, but the fact of turning to Ben as mentor turned Shane sour.

The doctor made a weekly check of the cast and even specified a date when it could come off. This caused cheer in Tim's camp. He would train within reason still and stretch his body to keep limbered up and the lactic acid out of his used muscles. Each stretch caused a sensation of euphoria within the man. Tingling with triumph after a half hour series of yoga movements, Tim could begin his days wonderfully.

Shane, on the other hand, was getting wound up about the contact with Ben still. No good reason, mind, just hints and allusions. Allegations made by him, for him and it truly peeved off nobody else other than Shane.

He was maybe being a bit of a loser, a turkey, a donkey (stubborn in his opinions), a blinded youth – blind to the reality of a successful young ethics professor. Shane wanted to vent his frustration and he had nobody to take it out on. He was fed up with all that lonely masturbation. Shane wanted to be a somebody, a Nobel prize-winning scientist, although nobody else would propose him for such an accolade at this point in his life and career.

Tim would get on doing whatever it was he would do, whether that would mean sit-ups, jogging a circuit, assisting Sainsbury's management, researching his sport, or offering consolation to Claire Morris. He was not necessarily looking to strike a chord with Suzanna though.

She would hold her head high, full of optimism. Her mother would call her 'Pollyanna', as she believed that her daughter had no grasp of reality, anyway. She thought that she suffered a breach of contract in this way with life's truths.

Some mothers do have 'em? Yeah but what about mentioning the progeny who have those damned folk too, to boot, the kind of people who rearrange, or rummage, or shuffle about in a once perfectly ordered sequence of affairs. The biologists call it respecting boundaries. A physical necessity if anything of worth is to come about.

To boot a cockerel up the ass would be nothing for a farmer trying to collect eggs from the barn, so why then is it something for the day-visitor who dropped his camera? In this respect Shane would forgive himself the urge for wanting to cause physical damage to an opponent. He was indeed a black belt in a martial art and would not think too hard about using his skills if necessary. He hated with a vehemence some things in life.

Shane was something of a bad egg, really. Although he would train with Tim where possible and was a star athlete in his own right, he would take out his angst on experiments in the laboratory. Also, when in the Dojang three times a week Shane would sometimes utilise his talents against an opponent. He actually desired to fight at the Olympics too as a Taekwondo artist, but life would not see this happen. He was not Aaron Cook.

This fact (which he understood but couldn't bring himself to admit) and his grossly ambitious science-life caused an inner tension that amounted to volcanic flows such as Vesuvius or Etna or Popocatapetl erupting from within every now and again.

He was a bit of a dangerous character in all. Nobody could tell that just by looking. Suzanna had hinted at it, and their parents knew that something was not quite right. Maybe it was the marijuana he had smoked at a party some months before. Maybe it was his lack of success at sexual conquesting. He was getting fed up with it all. Shane knew what he wanted but couldn't have it.

Some things in this life were simply out of reach. And for those who get them, well, they probably deserved it and worked hard to get it. In this case, blind ambition was ruling his mind. All his fitness and knowledge combined led him to the conclusion that his self-worth was far in excess of his current position. Shane was losing his patience and his Sensei would not hear of this. After all, the disciplines of Self-respect, Integrity, Honesty, Fitness, and Justice were integral to the world of Taekwondo.

Shane was his own star, and he wanted to be the world's superstar, as do many young achievers. Only, some pressures were mounting and he was losing control a little.

Tim was in on this. He already had been involved in helping Claire Halls rehabilitate earlier on. Would it be fair on him that he dived in for Shane too? After all, they were training buddies. And maybe they knew too much about each other already just to let things slip all of a sudden.

Suzanna got on in Collage. Tim got on in Sainsburys. Shane got on in the Physics Laboratory. And sure enough, three weeks later the cast came off and he could begin swimming once again; and cycling too(easy now).

Benjamin Williams was thoroughly enraptured by his new role as a mentor to a potential Olympic medallist. How would the season conclude now, then? Tim had maintained sufficient fitness throughout the three weeks on the exercise bike. Although tempted to go out on a drinking bender to drown his temporary blues away, he kept his composure; and with Ben's new-found guidance trained some more.

In truth, his arm still hurt. It twinged a little. Especially with any sudden movements. The good Doctor had advised him not to swing, punch, arm-wrestle, shake loose, or otherwise distort a weakened wrist. This seemed to make good sense to Tim. He would still use Ben's exercise bike twice a week in the mornings, and exercise a yoga routine three times a week.

Some would find his yoga somewhat unconventional. Some people found it all together weird that he would do this type of exercise. "Sod 'em! Stuff them! Get off my freight train, you bitches," Tim would say.

His struggle was now on. Could he get to the trials and make good in May? There were just four months to go. The breakage had occurred in November and the cast came off in December, leaving him with the super-trial challenge of rising like a Phoenix from the flames. "The Phoenix lives, baby - the Phoenix lives - You will see." Tim hollered at some passing traffic after a particularly fine training session.

Basically he had motivation. Nothing or nobody could take this away from him. He was a wonder to marvel at. Tim, the astronomer's new discovery; Tim, the astrologer's find. He was on a different planet to the others. He required competition and competition required him.

He was on the way to the London 2012 Olympics and to a place in athletic history. Only time would tell, only time would differentiate whether or not he could win on the day. Time would be the mother of all healers, the father of all purpose.

Tim was still very young and had time on his side. This could only be a good thing. Tim's struggle had really only just begun. A fractured wrist would not stand in his way after all, a stressed out training partner would not prevent an inevitable rise to furtherance from occurring. He would strive, and in so striving, become; and in so becoming, be born again – every time.

There was something of a constant Renaissance about him. Every day would spell out a new beginning, a day of differentials and challenges unbetold. An unwinding of some periphery or other; an unfolding of constant mystery. Life was a miracle, and in Tim's case, a miracle worth living. He would see to it alright.

He could have planted a traffic cone on his best friend's doorstep and got clean away with it. Nobody would think to hassle Tim over such an incident. Anyway, he probably wouldn't be planting any traffic cones at all, just the thought that this sort of thing happens on a daily basis in any locality in the UK.

Tim had hunger, 'tiene hambre' as they say in Spanish. Or in French 'Il a le faim d'un loup', he had the hunger of a wolf. This equated to his prowess more so than at the dinner table. Although, I'm sure that if asked he would gladly request extra pasta, potatoes, or beans. This would equate to a great appetite. He was a force for good, a leader amongst his peers, a creator – not a destroyer, a man who was attempting to defy the odds and set new standards on a regular basis. Each meeting was a new opportunity to do so. He was dedicated. Dedicated to incremental improvement.

He had learnt from the greats of our universe that the only true favour that one can ever do for oneself is to make personal improvements every day, no matter how large or how small. In this way, if every human being on a cricket team made an improvement of 1% every day, that's a net efficiency improvement of 11% in a single day, and 77%in a single week! The team that was to promote such a rate of improvements would surely win the Ashes.

Tim had learnt that every member of the British rugby team was classed as clinically obese by the medical board. Their muscle-to-bone-to-body-fat ratio would outweigh the average height-weight ratio for a typical adult male. Tim was smart enough to realise that this information, though based on scientific research, was not necessarily the ultimate order of the day.

He always took note when it came to physically life-changing discoveries. He would need to be honed for an optimal performance after all.

So the struggle was on. The struggle to stay slim, the struggle to keep his cool, to keep his head on his shoulders and feet on the ground. The struggle for survival in an ultra-competitive community of athletes. Would he be overshadowed or even outclassed by others in his class?

What a dull life. 'All work and no play made Jack a very dull kid, indeed', said Jack Nicholson. Tim was indeed a hard worker, with morale, ethics, values and principles. He had no social life beyond his training partnership with Shane and Suzanna, beyond his philanthropic relationship with Claire Morris, and student-mentorship with Benjamin Williams. He knew Alex Davies from visiting Collage from time to time with the crew, but would keep fairly quiet upon visiting.

Nobody complained. People just respected that his talents required daily toning. He had a whole heap of support from family and friends. Tim was valued, both on the course and as a close associate. He may not have realised it at the time, but he had people wanting to step into his shoes and race with equal dexterity.

Kids would shout encouraging remarks as he flew past. "Go get 'em, tiger!" or "Rock on, Tommy!" Clearly, not everyone actually knew his name at this stage, so it was still up in the air, but they just knew that he was good at what he was doing.

"You're all balls and ass" commented one observer meaning that he had a lot of courage and strong legs. Tim continued.

Suzanna was by now having family discussions about her brother Shane. She was worried. Shane was a bit scary from time to time. He meant well by her. He only wanted to be her protector, but maybe his ideals had been stretched too far, beyond what was or would be real. He meant to stand in, to ward off any unwarranted suitor. Perhaps he hadn't thought that Suzanna may desire a suitor. In fact she still rather fancied her chances with Tim. Ben made advances which were not rejected, but Shane made it terribly difficult.

She was young, too, with thoughts and feelings. Her brother was perhaps a little messed up, though. Anyway, one way or another the situation would arrange itself for the better in the long run. Tim, truth being told, had primitive urges towards her. This was both unspoken and not acted upon. In the guise of concentrating on the forthcoming Games.

They would all resolve their personal predicaments by means of meeting some external criteria, thus taking the mental process off of the libidinous lustfulness that drove so many to eternal damnation. Tim had faith in God. Maybe this was what made him so strong. He would often attend church on a Sunday morning to make a tithing. He did not take this lightly and made humble reverences whenever he could.

Some days, Tim would just feel like talking to God and would go off to some quiet place to sit and pray, meditate or cogitate. Maybe his true struggle would be in finding a place close to God. Perhaps his whole life paled into insignificance alongside the Almighty. Tim the wonderful, becoming Tim the humbled-one.

Either way, Tim had truly discovered that each new day would bring about challenges untold, ideas unheard of, and faith to carry it through. Tim's struggle was truly just commencing.

Chapter 13
Triathlon Days

"So tell us about your grandpa, Tim."
"What kind of a man was he?"
"How come he got to the Olympics?"

The questions came flooding in, and Tim just knew that he would be obliged to answer them. At least, some, anyway.

Grandpa Billy was a fit man and had made it into his seventies. The Richardson family enjoyed celebrating his life. He had been an achiever, a sportsman of the first class, and a family man.

Grandpa Billy had participated in the 1960 Rome Summer Olympic Games in the marathon, at the age of 26, and had ran well in a time of 2hours 18 minutes. Unbeknown to Billy, his wife-to-be had been travelling in Italy at that exact time and was touring round then. They would meet in later years back on English soil and both have a tremendous story to tell.

Grandpa Billy was a disciplined man. He kept a strict regime of diet, exercise, psychology, and meditation throughout his entire Olympic days. Tim went on to explain to them that he remembered his Grandpa's earliest wish.

That was that a member of his family should return to the Olympics again one day. Tim could vividly recall being sat around the television with Grandpa Billy as they watched numerous races from the Games in the 1990s, including the Commonwealth Games, European and World Championships, and the Olympic Games. Tim was born feeling inspired by the man.

In a nutshell, Grandpa Billy had seasoned him from the word 'Go!' to get out there and reach for the stars.

Tim went on reflecting about his Olympic Grandpa for some time, until everyone's questions had been answered or at least entertained.

Then somebody asked "Why did you choose the Trek Madone for your cycling, buddy?"

Tim replied. "You're quite right, my bike is a Trek Madone 4.0. It costs over £3,000 new, but I got lucky with part-sponsorship, part-savings as well."

He continued "My options were fourfold: Cannondale, Claud Butler, Giant, or Trek."

A comic amongst them spoke up "Guys, don't worry, everything's alright, my bike's a Claud Butler!" It seemed funny in an abstract way that Geoff had suddenly said so.

Tim continued "I had a love affair with this Trek Madone 4.0. I saw it in the magazine and researched on the internet. Lance Armstrong won at least one of his world-famous Tour de France victories on this model bike. All feedback came in positive. I had to have it. I had to get this baby!"

Suzanna coerced "I agree…I reckon that I could beat you if we swapped bikes you know?"

"Yeah right; we'll see about that one Suze."

Tim talked bikes and technical stuff for some time, then they got onto the topic of times and distances.

"What's the quickest triathlon you've ever completed Tim?"

"That would depend on the distance. They range from Super-Sprint, to Sprint, to Olympic distance, to half IronMan, to full IronMan come to that."

"Go on – how far are they?"

"That varies from a 250m swim, 5km bike ride and 2.5km run to a 500m swim, 10km bike ride and 5km run, to Olympic distance swim 1500m, bike 40km and run 10km. And then you get your IronMan which goes crazy…swimming for 4 miles, cycling 150km and running a marathon (42km). I would love to do IronMan Hawaii one day, that's my dream, that's on the cards."

"You're crazy, you know that?"

"Say what you want, I know where I'm at."

"You're stark raving mad Tim. Anybody who swims 4 miles, cycles 150km and then runs a marathon is clearly off their trolly!"

"Yeah, yeah…I don't care. IronMan Hawaii here I come. I'll see you at the end with a Pina Colada, a grass skirt, and a hoola dancer."

"You're funny. At least you still have a sense of humour buddy."

"Tell us about your BMX Tim. Why don't you ride your BMX so much these days?" asked one member.

"What kind of BMX did you first buy?" asked another.

"My first BMX was a Univega, a present from Mum and Dad, with front and rear stunt pegs. This provided hours of entertainment. I learnt to wheelie, endo, spin and croggy on this bike."

"I got serious when I turned 15…wanted to buy a Diamondback. There were no sponsors at this point so I spent a year saving up £175 for a Diamondback BMX bike."

He continued, "Mum and Dad were furious. They had bought me the Univega for Christmas as a gift. They were peeved at me, man were they half."

"Sounds like your parents really care for you then Tim."

"Yeah – they do support me."

Tim, Suzanna and the boys talked bikes and triathlons for a whole afternoon before Suzanna decided it was time to train some more. "Sunday training; 220 or under, is the time to get for me. You can bet your bottom dollar if I got that time I would get sponsors too you know. Raaaaa!"

She guffawed after that outburst.

Tim, being the star, had the final say in the matter of triathlon. He agreed to go right ahead and do some running with her and her brother Shane. Geoff had to go off to so some homework.

So the three got changed, drank some Lucozade Sport drink, stretched, and set out for a 10km jog together on Sunday evening. The next race was due to come up in two weeks time.

With that in mind, Tim set his sights on winning, again! Shane had his sights on a top 25 finish, and Suzanna on gaining a pb at the event. There were due to be over 200 people competing at the event, participating in various distances, but approximately 85 in the Olympic distance race which Tim would be in.

Tim could feel the adrenalin pumping – his main competitor, Jonathan Bateman may just pip him to the post. He was known for his sprint finishes and his amazing endurance on the bike ride.

Nothing could stand in the way of his training. Even his supervisors at J Sainsbury's would not be able to prevent his early mornings and evening-time training sessions. Tim had focus, he had belief, and he had the physiology to prove it. He was on track and heading for the Games.

His mentor Ben, would try to steer clear out of his way, but would matter of factly ply him full of wisdom, sagacity, and Olympic knowledge – where the Games were, who participated, who won medals, the political movements of the day – referring to the boycotts, such as the 1980-1984 Cold War between the USA and the then USSR, or the Moscow and Los Angeles Games respectively; or the demonstrations around the world prior to the 2008 Beijing Games.

Also, the lucky mascots used symbolically, the economies: national, global and local, the Presidents, the Prime Ministers, the fuel, the drive, the energy, the passions that lead the way. Tim was awash with historical context about the Games because of Ben. Ben was an expert in the matter. He had done his homework.

Tim regarded Tim Don as something of a demi-God, since he had won the World Championship; and Alistair Brownlee as superhuman since he had run in the Beijing Games. In truth, he was a king of physique, psychology and speed. Alistair could make the fittest seem sluggish, the fastest seem beat, the leanest and the meanest seem downwind. He ruled the roost and Tim wanted to step right up into his shoes. He wanted his footwear; all of his achievements had been catalogued and compiled into Tim's athletic scrapbooks. He had been following him over the last three years as a long term project. Now Tim was determining to have him beat.

Tim was willing to step up his own game and see to it that the 'boss man' be felled.

By the time their 10km run was finished, Tim, Shane, and Suzanna were planning their next training session together. A Monday morning swim and a Tuesday evening bike ride. The intensity between these three was high whilst they trained. They just knew that something big was afoot; some potential news for the world to report on. Ever determined, Tim moved on.

They decided to meet at the café for a breakfast fruit smoothie in the morning. Suzanna had this thing about cafés. She enjoyed the social aspect as much as the beverage itself.

She knew that she needed Alex in this respect. She also contained a secret. She fancied Tim, but dare not let on for fear of it ruining their training schedule. Also, there was the thing with Ben. Ben wanted to go out with her – probably more – but her brother was not having any of this. Shane still considered Ben to be unworthy of his sister's hand. He hated Ben because of this.

The three athletes, however, were a clique. They had plans – Shane, Suzanna and Tim. They had plans, yes Sir, they had plans together. Mainly to send Tim to the London 2012 Games.

Ben was a spanner in the works for liking Suzanna. Shane would tell him "Feel free to profess your ethicals dude, but don't come near my sister, OK!"

A plan foiled. The catch – Ben was both old enough and wise enough to be dating girls by now, Suzanna knew that. She actually had no qualms in explaining that to her brother.

There was a fight in the air. Ben knew he had to persevere. Like the lottery he thought – "one shouldn't give up just because one doesn't win on the first attempt." Ben also knew that if it came to the crunch, Shane would probably win, being the athlete n' all. But he had no fear. He decided to stick to his guns and persist with Suzanna.

As the days rolled by, Ben continued to plan how he might make further advances on Suzanna. Shane began to conspire – how could he demonstrate he was protecting his sister?

Ben continued to teach at college, all the while holding a full-time job, mentoring Tim, and looking after Pépé. Shane grew jealous of his accomplishments. His animosity had begun to grow rife.

Unfortunately for Ben, the first real untoward event of his entire life was about to unfold. Ben was a mature man in his late twenties. His brain, his mind was ahead of his peers. He was a very intelligent chap. He had the respect from other college professors and his students listened to his words.

Anyhow, the crunch came one afternoon whilst Ben had chosen to personally visit Suzanna at her home. He had decided to try again, only from a different angle. What a mistake that turned out to be.

Ben arrived at the door and she answered.

"Hello."
"Hello."
"I came to see you"
"Oh, OK – I don't think you should really – probably not a great idea."
"No, it's OK. Really. There are some things that I would like to say."
"Well come in for five minutes. Shane is not home right now."

They went into the kitchen and Ben began to tell her how much he liked her and that they should get together sometime for coffee, a movie, or a concert. She went along with this with an open-mind, and suddenly the front door opened.

"Suze, I'm home!" yelled Shane.
"Oh no – " said Suzanna.
Continuing, she said "Quick Ben, you'd better leave now."

Ben was in no hurry to leave however. By this time the two young men were face to face in the kitchen. You could sense the anger, the instant karmic shift from Shane.

Silence for quite a moment. Then he spoke.

"I thought I told you not to come near my sister?"
"It's cool. Don't worry."
"No – it's far from cool. Not only have you ignored my words, you've also set foot in my own kitchen."

Silence again.

Ben got rude suddenly "Shut the fuck up." Aside to Suzanna he said "What a moron."

Shane snapped "What did you just say? What did you call me?"

"I think you heard."

Shane boiled red with indignation. He reached for Ben and grabbed him by the collar. He started yelling.

"You steer clear now you understand. Go back to your Greek and your school children – asshole!"

Continuing he screamed: "Stay the hell away from my sister!"

Ben pushed him away, hard.

Shane shouted "That's it - I don't care."

With that he grabbed a kitchen knife and began gesticulating in a menacing fashion, threatening all the while. He repeatedly yelled "I don't care!"

Then, suddenly, Shane slammed the knife down on the kitchen counter and Suzanna uttered quietly "I think you should leave now Ben." She had screamed when Shane had picked up the knife "Don't Shane, don't be stupid!" That's probably why he put it down again.

Ben left the room and the house. He walked away feeling bitter once again. He would run the situation over again and again in his mind before returning to his beloved Pépé. Ben had tried again, against expectation and had failed – at least in the immediate term anyway.

Back in the kitchen Shane and Suzanna were arguing furiously. She couldn't quite grasp that Shane was either that stupid or jealous. Ben had the credentials. Shane had the ambitions. They really didn't see eye to eye.

"How are we supposed to train together with this going on?"

"You're so stupid Shane. Ben's no harm and now look what you've gone and done."

Shane's mood swings were beginning to concern Suzanna, but the argument cooled off once again and Shane went out in a huff.

Ben had simply returned home, reflecting all the while. He felt a bit shaken by the event but not too badly.

***

Some time passed and it came to the day of the race two weeks later. There was Tim, Shane and Suzanna all clubbed together to win the race and achieve best times and places respectively.

Tim was wearing a red and grey Asics tracksuit over his swimwear and some Asics gel Cumulus trainers. He knew the motto "Anima

Sana In Corpore Sano" in Latin, meaning "a sound mind in a sound body".

To begin with he would have to swim 1500 metres in his Speedo swimsuit. Then the changeover. He would have 200 metres to strip out of the wetsuit and put on his Pearl Izumi cycling shoes, and pedal 40km as fast as possible on his Trek Madone 4.0. Then the final haul, yet another changeover and a 10km run in his Asics trainers.

Tim had his sights firmly on winning as did his sponsors for him. A win would mean a definite place on Team GB. Would he be able to perform?

Shane and Suzanna prepared for their races too. Both had the fitness, both fully prepared for another triathlon to take place. They had eaten a lot of spaghetti the night before and were now munching on bananas and energy gels to prepare themselves further. All the training could be said to have paid off. Here in Ripon the annual event was about to begin.

Ben was hovering around amongst the spectators. Tim knew he was there but didn't wish to spark off a further feud with Shane. He had been told all about it.

As time drew nearer to the event, tracksuits came off, goggles went on, stretches occurred, deep breathing, mental focusing, and the thought of the prize money for the winner. A cheque for £250 1st place, £125 2nd place, and £50 3rd place was up for grabs. A handsome bounty as ever.

Suddenly they were underway. The ladies race set off half an hour ahead of the gents. Suzanna felt brave enough to set her own pace in the swim. Arms were flailing everywhere. She wore a nose clip though to prevent her from inhaling water up her nose. This would be a distraction from the swimming. She felt comfortable at that pace and knew from the training that she could get a good time at that speed.

Half an hour later Tim and Shane raced for the water. They began – Tim kicked straight off amongst the leaders, Shane shortly behind.

The pace was very fast indeed. Tim was in fifth place after the swimming, Shane back in 22nd.

Then the transition came about, the tough part, the change of footwear and the stripping of swimwear; all very quick, very adept.

Suzanna was feeling strong. She hopped onto her bike (a Cannondale racer) and made powerful piston-like pedals right away. She was in good motion.

Shane had received a punch to the head whilst swimming and a kick to the chest. He soldiered on though.

Tim got straight to the crunch. On the bike and regaining positions quickly – 4th and then 3rd. He could see Jonathon Bateman in 2nd place and felt the tactic upon him. Stay on his tail until the run. Take him over if possible. Whenever possible. Somebody, unbeknown to Tim, was currently leading the race. Ah? What exactly would he do about that?

He raced. He powered. He breathed. He envisaged winning. He couldn't bare the thought of not winning this important meet. So Tim kept on Bateman's tail for 25km. Then suddenly – wings! He flew. He had the vibe. He overtook Jonathon Bateman and into 2nd place. The leader was in his sights now. Not far to go. He felt confident that when it came to the run he would regain his rightful position.

Shane battled on. Sticking in the top 25 was his prerogative.

The run, the 10km stretch. Tim could belt round in under 35 minutes – tried and tested. He had done countless times before. Why not today once again? No reason at all why not. The Charge of the Light Brigade. He had drank his Lucozade Sport alright. Wings once again. He ran like the wind. Speed of light. All the while catching the number one dude, catching, catching, catching, catching, and level by the 4km marker. 6km to go.

Suzanna never battered an eyelid. Totally unflustered with her own stride, the race was on. She was comfortable with her own pace, though simultaneously pushing herself to a new limit.

Tim was now leading the race. All his heart, all his lungs, all his legs. He was pounding the street. His soul was bursting. He had to win. The timer vehicle continued right in front of him so he could check the time. 3km, 2km, 1km to go. He had made good time. He could hear the loudspeaker hail him in.

"Coming in as this year's champion at the Ripon Triathlon is number 127 Mr Tim Richardson. Let's hear it everybody. What a fine specimen of an athlete!"

And with that, Tim made a final 100 metre dash and crossed the line. He had done it. He had won the race, the first prize and a place on Team GB as a consequence. He was fit, but exhausted.

Ben went wild. He applauded and gesticulated in the air with a victorious fist. "Yeah!"

As the rest of the athletes progressed, Suzanna achieved a personal best time and Shane – though a little battered from the swim – appeared in 24th position. All missions accomplished.

Ben forgot himself and went to see Tim. He was delighted. An outstanding achievement as ever.

These Triathlon Days were good days; exciting. What a success. Ben had been a key player. Tim constantly recognised this.

Shane took a hot shower and put on some dry clothes. Suzanna came over to check Tim's result and gave a whoop of triumph for him.

They were on the way. If Tim could pull this off again in London they were the team. They would be made.

The ceremony was fun. Tim received his medal and Jonathon Bateman had come in 3rd place just behind the mystery athlete in 2nd. Two gorgeous young girls pecked him on the cheek and handed him his cheque.

Tim was a happy camper. He had done it again.

Chapter 14
Benjamin's theorem

Ben figured that Esperanto had the potential to help the entire world. Founded by 'Dr Esperanto' Ludwig Zamenhof, a Polish optician, and first published in 1887, the language knew no barriers. Offically, this language was multi-cultural, but not of any country or ethnic group. It was a neutral, international language.

With over 2 million speakers around the world in most countries, the language consisted of over 100,000 words, of which 20,000 acted as root words. The literal translation of the word 'Esperanto' means 'one who hopes'. With this in mind, and being an Esperanto speaker himself, Ben did have his hopes.

Ben saw beauty in the simplicity of the language and figured that, just as Franz Kafka once said, "Anyone who keeps the ability to see beauty never grows old". He had made countless contacts over the years with natives of many countries from as far afield as China, Japan, Russia, or Taiwan. Closer to home, he sometimes spoke the language to a French contact.

Ben agreed with the maxim that a tiny pebble could cause great ripples – the law of cause and effect, action and reaction. Esperanto was his pebble, and the world his pond in which to throw it. Not that there weren't others already doing exactly this.

Esperanto was an acorn to Ben, about to grow into a Great Oak; the flap of the wings of a butterfly in the Amazon rainforest about to cause a tidal wave in Malaysia. He saw sense and direction in the language, such a simple concept that stood to gain believers, save millions in translation costs, and create a sense of unity in a world of unrest.

With a library full of literature, a music hall full of recording artists, annual conventions and radio broadcasts, the idea seemed to be onto a winner. Translations into Esperanto could be seen to range from: Hemingway's 'The Old Man and the sea', Tolkien's 'The Lord of the Rings', Garcia Marquez's 'One Hundred Years of Solitude',

'The Holy Bible', Umar Khayyam's 'Rubaiyat', Grass's 'The Tin Drum', Marco Polo's 'Book of Wonders', Cao Xuequin's ' Dream of the Red House' – a great family saga, and for children, Asterix the Gaul, TinTin, Winnie-the-Pooh, Strewelpeter, Pippi Longstocking, the complete Moomintroll books of world-renowned Finnish author Tove Jansson, as well as the Oz books of L. Frank Baum. Translations out of Esperanto include Maskerado – a book published in 1965 by Tivadar Soros (father of the financier George Soros) detailing the survival of his family during the Nazi occupation of Budapest. This book can be found in English, US American, Russian, German, and Turkish.

The flourishing literary tradition in Esperanto has been recognised by PEN International, which accepted an Esperanto affiliate at its 60th Congress in September 1993. Notable present-day writers in Esperanto include the novelists Trevor Steele (Australia), Istvan Nemere (Hungary), and Spomenka Stimec (Croatia); the poets William Auld (Scotland), Mikhail Gishpling (Russia/Israel) and Abel Montagut (Catalonia); and the essayists and translators Probal Dasgupta (India), Fernando de Diego (Venezuala) and Kuisu Kei (Japan). Auld was nominated for the Nobel Prize in Literature in both 1999 and 2000 for his contribution to poetry.

More than a hundred international conferences and meetings are held each year in Esperanto, without translators or interpreters. The biggest is the World Congress of Esperanto, held in Adelaide (1997), Montpellier (1998), Berlin (1999), Tel-Aviv (2000), Zagreb (2001), Fortaleza, Brazil (2002), Gothenburg, Sweden (2003), Beijing, China (2004), and Vilnius, Lithuania (2005). The first symposium of Esperanto speakers in Arab countries took place in Amman in 2000. The fifth All-Americas Congress was held in Mexico City in 2001, and afterwards, the Asian Congress in Seoul in 2002.

Ben was particularly impressed with the language as many musicians had recorded in Esperanto as well. Musical genres in the language included popular and folk songs, rock, cabaret, solo, choir pieces and opera. Popular composers and performers, including Britain's Elvis Costello and the USA's Michael Jackson, recorded in Esperanto, or used it in their promotional materials.

Several tracks from the all-Esperanto Warner Music album Esperanto, launched in Spain in November 1996, were placed high on the Spanish pop charts. Classical orchestral and choral pieces with texts in Esperanto include Lou Harrison's La Koro Sutro, and David Gaine's first symphony, both from the US. Ben had heard recordings of these and could appreciate where they were coming from. Music in Esperanto could be found on-line, including several sites devoted to Esperanto karaoke.

Plays by dramatists as diverse as Goldoni, Ionesco, Shakespeare, and Scarborough's very own Alan Ayckbourn, have been performed in recent years in Esperanto. A production of Shakespeare's King Lear was put on in Hanoi, Vietnam, recently, with a local cast. Although Chaplin's The Great Dictator used Esperanto-language signs in its sets, feature-length films were less common. A notable exception, however, could be William Shatner's Incubus, whose dialogue was entirely in Esperanto.

Radio stations in Austria, Brazil, China, Cuba, Estonia, Hungary, Italy and Poland broadcasted regularly in Esperanto, as did Vatican Radio. Several programs were also available over the Internet. TV stations in various countries broadcasted Esperanto courses, including a recent 16-part adaptation of the BBC's Muzzy in Gondoland on the Polish Channel One network.

Ben realised that Esperanto was designed to be spoken as a 'second language', not as a 'mother-tongue'. He hoped that more people would accept the language for what it was. He suffered at the hands of the critics, and was known as an eccentric because of his belief in a minority global language, although anybody could see that because Esperantists were dispersed around the world, the language was capable of uniting people who spoke dramatically different languages (eg Chinese and Mexicans), including those who did not necessarily speak English well, if at all.

He had researched on the Internet and discovered chat rooms, clubs, dissemination of scientific papers, novels, science-fiction, poetry, and more. He understood from this that electronic networks were the fastest-growing means of communication amongst Esperantists. With more than several hundred mailing lists for discussions ranging from family-use of language, to the Theory of Relativity, Esperanto was widely used in chatrooms.

Some of the other professors at Scarborough Campus doubted whether Ben's beliefs would ever pay off. Not being a national language, critics doubted the usefulness of this man-made language. Compared to, say Lithuanian, Latvian, Estonian, or Tongan (2 million speakers each), these national languages could be said to be less useful than Esperanto as the only speakers are concentrated in one geographical region.

Ben knew full well from reading C S Lewis that 'the future is something which everyone reaches at the rate of sixty minutes an hour, whatever he does, whoever he is'. The future of Esperanto was still bright; over one hundred years in and still ticking. He had hope, and in talking to some global colleagues, he could see full well that this language stood in good soil. With the right nurturing, this acorn could still grow.

Come what may, whether or not Ben continued believing, contacting, communicating, writing, speaking, or walking his own talk, he could quote a very wise Australian, Andrew Matthews, who once said that "the universe has no favourites; it rains on rich and poor alike. The same universal laws apply to each and every one of us". Ben figured that though small and rained upon by the cynics, Esperanto would one day see the sunshine and grow into a great titan of global significance.

Ben knew that the effective communication of the language depended very much on the 5 "W's" of communication – Who? (source) says What? (message) in What Way? (channel) to Whom? (receiver) and with What Effect? (feedback). He had hopes on being the right person with the right message, in the right place, at the right time. Armed with this ambition he cared very little for the insults of his parochial, English-speaking work colleagues.

Interestingly enough, every year, one or two of his students would express an interest in learning the language, or at least to find out a little more about the goings-on of Esperanto and its followers. He lost no time at all in directing them to his collection of Esperanto magazines – 'Monato', and 'Fonto', two of over 100 magazines and journals published regularly in the language.

Ben had actually formulated a plan on how best to market Esperanto. He had selected a target market in his mind, and hoped to follow through with this over the coming years, using his post as a launch-pad for his ideas. Ranging from linguists, students and teachers/lecturers, to political leaders and the United Nations, he had the idea that people with an active passion for languages would be all potentially liable to be intrigued about the prospects of Esperanto.

Open-minded young people with everything to learn and the whole world in which to learn it would be second-to-none for him. He knew from his own job that professors had the power to communicate important lessons to students of all ages, thus influencing future generations by conducting classes, seminars, lectures and so forth. Politicians, vested with the power to influence entire nations and to shape a country, would be in a strong position to accept, appreciate and further the language.

As for the United Nations, a typical meeting with, say, people from 21 countries speaking 21 languages, would require translations going thousands of different ways. The translation costs would be astronomical, and what's more, complete and accurate translations would be very difficult to come by. However, were Esperanto implemented – the International Language – suddenly costs would be tumbling exponentially, and all translations would be understood on a level-footing.

Multi-National Corporations involve many overseas branches – eg HSBC, Starbucks, BMW, Wal-Mart/Asda, Jaguar, Merril Lynch, Barclaycard, Glaxo-SmithKline, Toyota, or Lexus for example – and the language barriers thus presented require employees to be multi-lingual with at least two fluent languages in order to conduct business efficiently. Esperanto, in this medium, would facilitate the whole communication arena. Deals between Russia and China have been struck and fully documented in Esperanto, for example.

Anybody watching a movie could appreciate that this medium is a powerful and important means of communicating messages to viewers. By using Esperanto in film, many other people would become aware of the benefits involved and purpose to it.

Ben had invented a slogan for his own communications... 'Esperanto – with a little hope comes a lot of scope'. Put so simply it turned no heads, but those who came across it could appreciate its meaning. He had a big idea to publish a British newspaper in Esperanto on a daily basis, alongside all the other foreign papers. If people saw this on the shelves he figured that heads would surely pick up and pay attention.

As for advertising and the promotion plan, Ben reckoned that word-of-mouth communication could cause many people's initial interest in the language. Media interviews with Esperantists and subsequently publishing the dialogue would demonstrate this. A journalist's fees may range upwards of £50/article, newspapers ranging from 60 pence to £1.40 / product, therefore many £thousands changing hands on a daily basis.

He knew from the congresses that advertising the slogans on mugs, keyrings, balloons, calendars, business cards, t-shirts, pens etc would be a cause of Direct Marketing, available to all attendees. On a grander scale, billboards, buses, world wide web, metros, TV commercials, and radio jingles could appeal to a wider audience.

What would be the costs of all this? Well, Ben reckoned that a teacher could charge upwards of £25/hour, merchandise sold at a reasonable rate eg £5/mug, £.80/pen, £6/t-shirt, £12/CD, £8/book, £6/cinema ticket, £150/billboard advert, £500/bus advert etc.

The language had been freely evolving since its inception in the year 1887. Rapidly growing in one century from one man's private invention to well over two million speakers. No need to spend years in school learning numerous national languages when you could learn Esperanto in just a fraction of the time. Suddenly 'Global Village' took on a whole new meaning. Not just the world-wide-web, but Esperanto would take the concept to a whole new level.

The Universal Esperanto Association (UEA), whose membership forms the most active part of the Esperanto community, has national affiliates in 62 countries, and individual members in almost twice that number. There were especially notable concentrations of speakers in countries as diverse as China, Japan, Brazil, Iran, Hungary, Bulgaria, and Cuba. Numbers of textbooks sold each year were well into their hundreds of thousands.

With all this information in mind, Ben just had to reach out and share the joys of the language with his students. Some were more receptive than others. Occasionally, a smart-aleck would heckle him, stating that the world already had a global language and that was English; "Everybody speaks English already – are you mad?"

He had no qualms about making a stand for his beliefs and teaching on and around the subject in many ethical ways. The combination of Ethics and Esperanto seemed to go down particularly well in his mind. It would put his mind at ease when a student would come to him with a question about this language. The reward was there every now and again.

Just as a beautiful pearl is formed from the sand irritating the oyster on a constant basis, the evolution and progression of this magnificent International Language depended on the critics. After all, they were still within the bounds of an advert by so much as making mention of the topic.

Ben had plans to attend an annual congress at some point not too far away. He had been saving up and now that Pépé was around it would mean somebody looking after his dog for a week or so when he went. "No estas neniu kiel hundaĉo", he thought.

"Mia nomo estas Ben Williams, kaj mi kapablas okazigi ĉi tion, Esperanton," he made an oath to himself.

"La Junaj Trezor-serĉantoj" – Ben reflected 'what a cracking story book – The Young Treasure-Hunters – and they found it eventually, too. Took a bit of searching, but they got there in the end' - the childhood adventures of Katrina, Paulo, Georgo, and Anica, with Uncle Henriko in the background looking after them all.

Pépé was at his feet, lying down in the ground minding his own business and making groaning and farting noises every now and again. 'Tricky-woo got flop -bott; better call Herriott' Ben told the dog as a precaution. His warning had no effect on Pépé, though, and the dog just carried on doing what he always did in the first place, being a beast, a creature, a hunter's retrieving dog – originally bred for fetching birds back to the gunman, such as ducks on water, or grouse on the moor, pheasants or partridges, too. Pépé was fast growing up and no longer a puppy dog.

Although Ben was no hunter by nature, he went for walkies on a regular basis and gave the dog anti-worming tablets every few weeks just to make sure, and by order of the vet as well. He was happy to have a purpose and to be able to hold his head high at work. He had the respect of his students and work colleagues, even though he received taunts from time to time. People admired him for holding his position well.

One of Ben's favourite quotes was 'make hay while the sun shines……fojnadu dum la suno brilas'. He liked to think that Esperantists could help the world……Esperanton-paralantoj regas la mondon!

In talking to Suzanna, who was something of a Christian, he had begun reading the Bible in Esperanto and sometimes recited passages for her, such as Genesis (Genezo – Unua Libro de Moseo):

1 En la komenco Dio kreis la ĉielon kaj la teron.
2 Kaj la tero estis senforma kaj dezerta, kaj mallumo estis super la abismo; kaj la spirito de Dio ŝvebis super la akvo.
3 Kaj Dio diris: estu lumo: kaj fariĝis lumo.
4 Kaj Dio vidis la lumon, ke ĝi estas bona: kaj Dio apartigis la lumon de la mallumo.
5 Kaj Dio nomis la lumon Tago, kaj la mallumon Li nomis Nokto. Kaj estis vespero, kaj estis mateno, unu tago.

He was enthralled by the possibilities. The more he read, the more he got into it. Bit by bit, day by day Ben had hope.

He had learnt a few songs in Esperanto as well, not least of which was Ten Green Bottles. Dek Boteloj – "Dek boteloj pendas de la mur, Dek boteloj pendas de la mur, kaj se akcidente falus unu nur, Tiam nau boteloj pendus de la mur."

So on through ok, sep, ses kvin, kvar, tri, du, and then:

"Unu botelo pendas de la mur, Unu botelo pendas de la mur, Sed se akcidente falus unu nur, Tiam nur odoro pendus de la mur." (H W kaj N Holmes)

Another personal favourite for Ben was La Espero – music by F de Menil, lyrics by L L Zamenhof himself:

En la mondon venis nova sento,
Tra la mondo iras forta voko;
Per flugiloj de facila vento
Nun de loko flugu ĝi al loko.
Ne al glavo sangon soifanta
Ĝi la homan tiras familion:
Al la mond' eterne militanta
Ĝi promesas sanktan harmonion.

Sub la sankta signo de l'espero
Kolektiĝas pacaj batalantoj,
Kaj rapide kreskas la afero
Per laboro de la esperantoj.
Forte staras muroj de miljaroj
Inter la popoloj dividitaj:
Sed dissaltos la obstinaj baroj,
Per la sankta amo disbatitaj.

Sur neŭtrala lingva fundamento,
Komprenante unu la alian,
La popoloj faros en konsento
Unu grandan rondon familian.
Nia diligenta kolegaro
En laboro paca ne laciĝos,
Ĝis la bela sonĝo de l'homaro
Por eterna ben' efektiviĝos.

Ben would sing quietly to himself from time to time and encourage himself that it was all worthwhile. He had seen great potential in the language and thought that all school children ought to be taught the language from a very early age, as much to improve international relationships as anything else.

He spent time at college teaching and professing Ethics, so the language was a hobby for him, a private passion kept separate from his everyday job. Realising the benefits of such an endeavour to be extremely rewarding at the best of times, Ben continued with his career as well as branching out to spread the ramifications of the language.

His lectures at college would range in topic through corporate social responsibility, stakeholder theory of the firm, consequential theories – egoism, utilitarianism -, contemporary ethical theories – virtues, feminism, discourse ethics -, stakeholder relations, shareholders as stakeholders, employing people worldwide, sustainable consumption, suppliers and competitors as stakeholders, globalization (perfect cue for the impact and benefits of Esperanto), sustainability towards industrial ecosystems, and government regulation/business ethics.

He could talk at length about any aspect of his subject matter and had prepared much discourse on business ethics in particular. He particularly enjoyed looking into the influences on ethical decision-making, taking great pride in the wider perspective.

For Ben, his work would never be over. There was always something else to get his teeth stuck into, whether academic in nature, or something more personal and closer to his heart. There would always be something. He had found a great companion in Pépé. The dog was really making his day for him. Getting up in the morning and going out for a walk, feeding him at lunchtime and more exercise, then a trip round town to show him off to everybody else. That was the life for Ben and his doggo.

Pépé never minded about being shown off. He was a bit of a show off anyhow. Yapping and slobbering and rolling and chasing and jumping and sniffing and all the rest of it. Wholesome behaviour like this were the very essence of living for him and his master.

Whenever Ben would make contact with a new pen pal he would always send a photograph of himself with the dog. Everyone always commented on the friendly disposition as well. 'Kia hundo – what a dog!', they would say.

There was always an interest in his personal situation as well as professional circumstance from the contacts. "To be great is to be misunderstood," Ben would quote Emerson in reference to his personal take on his own greatness. Also, when a new student would seek his advice he would say, "When the student is ready, the teacher will appear".

This encouraged both and seemed to make good sense at the time. So this was Ben's theory, that Esperanto would rise in stature and one day become a global giant amongst all nations' languages. Membership had increased already from one man's private invention to an international community of millions. There were some big-time believers already in the world.

Fortunately for Pépé he needn't have worried either way, only caring for his next meal and when to go out for a walk. Loneliness thus dispelled, life seemed to be going places. Only, his heart still yearned for darling Suzanna. She was a busy bee as well with the café and triathlon training schedule.

How did she feel about Ben's theory? Intrigued would be one word for it, I guess. All things being said, the most enthused member of the 'crew' would have been Claire Morris (Linguist and musician). Her role had shifted so dramatically over the last few years from down and out to recording artist to mother to God knows what.

Ben had touched on the subject with her only once, or maybe twice, but her passion for foreign tongues was there, and the very word 'Esperanto' conjured up an aura of significance for her. Ben took delight in this.

Suzanna Jeffries had expressed an interest in the language, although not entirely captivated. She was more concerned with her own goals within the workplace and on the triathlon course. This seemed more real to her than a manmade language.

Anyhow, Ben was not to be dissuaded in any way. It was his support for this language that lead some of his colleagues to view him as a bit 'different' in some way. This did not perturb him. He valued Esperanto as an opportunity to travel the world. Almost a passport in itself, with the right contacts and correct application of linguistics, the world could be his oyster.

Ben was not advocating Esperanto for financial gain. His job paid a wage and he was happy with that, although a higher salary would have been useful to move to a bigger house in the suburbs, or to drive a more up-to-date car. However, he was able to afford his keep, and his girlfriend did not complain about chipping in every now and again.

They were through the worst patch. Shane had been blowing hot and cold over the years, a foolish, possessive behavioural pattern that could only lead to trouble if it continued. He needed to get out more. Ben had been his vent to release his angers, unfairly and unexpectedly at times, though the worst was now through with.

Shane had no interest in other languages. "Everybody speaks English. What's the point in learning other languages when the whole world already knows how to, or at least is learning how to, speak English? It is a self-fulfilling prophecy, if you ask me," he told Suzanna one day speaking on the topic.

"You're a cold-blooded snake, Shane. Think about others for a change, instead of it all being about me, me, me all the time," Suzanna scolded him.

She had been warming to Ben's theorem for a while and had come to accept that it had its merits. "We cannot change anything unless we first accept it," she quoted Carl Jung. "At least some people are trying to change the world out there. There is much territory out there, ground to be covered. Won't you just open your eyes, you dingbat", she reprimanded her brother again a little.

"I'm not getting into any of that with you, Suze. I am elsewhere right now and I don't need to know that kind of stuff, anyway. Who started this conversation in the first place?" Shane asked her.

"You are ungrateful you, you, you – oh never mind. Forget about it. Ben has a heart and you should know that," she went on. "And it's a good job that somebody round here does!"

Shane was more concerned with his Taekwondo schedule and physics lab than with any linguistics. He was not to be swayed however and the two siblings parted and went their separate ways for the day feeling bad about their argument.

They would make up again. They always did; just a bit of a turf war going on about who was right and who was wrong. This issue was more personal to Suzanna, who unbeknown to Ben, was seriously beginning to consider him for a partner by now.

This would be something of a revelation for future reference, bearing in mind that past performance is never a guarantee for future results to remain the same. In other words, her feelings for him might change, or grow, wax or wane, augment or diminish, rise or fall, an emotional harvest awaited.

Ben was never in the mood to physically assault anybody. He was a gentle soul with an awful lot of compassion for the human race. He was a firm advocate for peace in the world and could not stand the prospect of bloodshed and war. It all seemed so highly unethical to him. Hence he had become a professor and not a soldier.

He was glad that Suzanna had started to see him in a whole new light, a refreshing manner of sparks flying and a certain intangible magnetism between the two. Although they were more associates than anything else, there was always hope as far as Ben Williams was concerned.

He had his hopes pinned on a few things in life, but the most notable theory he entertained was his support of Esperanto. Professor Williams the wishful thinker, some would say about him. Professor Williams fighting a losing battle, others may have thought. He was not to be deterred.

Being interested in verse he sometimes could quote poetry as well:

Brilu, brilu eta stel',

Diamanto sur ĉiel'!
Diru kio estas vi,
Tiel alta super ni?

Kiam pasis taga glor',
Kaj la suno iris for,
Venas via lumigil',
Kara eta nokta bril'.

La maristo dankas vin,
Ĉar vi nokte gvidas lin.
Ĉu la vojon vidus li,
Se ne tiel brilus vi?

M C Butler

He enjoyed the poetry and treated it with due diligence and interest. Occasionally he would encourage his students to write their own poems, although that was extra-curricular. It was generally just the ethics that he focused on at college.

Ben was aware of a potential hazard, however. He figured that if a topic were to suffer significant apathy for an extended period of time, then the world would see the 'frog principle' in action. He feared that if not enough people kept the language alive then in time it would die out.

So what did this mean exactly, this frog principle? "Well," Ben began to explain his theory to a student, "if a frog is dropped into a pan of boiling hot water what will it do? Answer – it will try to jump out quickly. However, what if that same frog were dropped into a pan of pond water at natural temperature? Answer – not much, maybe swim around a little."

"But there is more" he continued, "if that same pan of pond water is gradually heated up, then what happens? Answer – the frog would not notice anything going on until it was too late. The water would become hot slowly and cook the frog."

His student asked how that fitted with Esperanto. "Well," Ben said, "if you viewed Esperanto as the frog and the world's national languages and native people as the water you could look at it in two different ways. Number one – the new language is destroyed by the already 'boiling hot' pre-existing languages and it gets squeezed out as people express no interest in this scheme. Or, number two – Esperanto is continually held at a small but steadily increasing level around the world. This would ensure that people know of its existence and the thought is always ticking away in the back of people's minds. By the time the water comes up to boiling point the language is a prepared and accepted part of culture today."

Ben had explained it as best he could, and it seemed to make sense to his student. "Oh, I get it," the student said. "It goes either way – either bad for the frog in which case he jumps out of the pan and the idea is rejected, or better for the frog in which case it gets cooked and people can eat it."

"Yes, the frog really has no choice in the matter....Esperanto already exists in the world and has done for over 120 years. Its destiny depends entirely on people's reaction to its value today and for the future."

"That's great," the student said. "Thankyou, Professor, I see it in a whole new light now."

With that the lesson concluded and Ben clasped and rubbed his hands together with glee at being able to spread the word to another human being. Small victories like this made it all seem worthwhile.

He certainly had his work cut out for him. No such thing as good luck or bad luck, just a steady evolution of events which may or may not be favourable. 'Steady Eddy', Ben thought of himself.

Regarding Suzanna, he knew not to get too attached. There was plenty of leeway for this relationship. A very wise Australian, Andrew Matthews, once said, "The moment you get too attached to things, people, money... you screw it up." Ben took note from these words to give a little break in between times. That is, in between meetings. These were not every week even, but often enough for now.

So, there was Benjamin's theory. Esperanto was onto a winner, though an underdog, manmade, and allegedly an 'artificial' language, Esperanto contained its own literature, music, media communications, governing body (the Universal Esperanto Association – UEA), movie scripts, plays, poetry, magazines, conferences, delegates, and many other annual events held the world over.

He personally supported this cause, with hope and aspirations for unity in the future. Professor Benjamin Williams, PhD : "Jen la mondo, personoj ŝatas esti kune. Esperanto povas kunvenigi la tutan mondon. Ĉiuj aŭskultu!"

Chapter 15
Apollo 13

"Houston, we have a problem!" Do you remember the brainstorming scene? The one where the space shuttle was hurtling rapidly out of control in outer space, due to lack of oxygen, and all the while the control team on planet earth were busy brainstorming how to build a new air vent out of a box, a tube and a very few other unlikely items. Well, they made it in the end before it was too late.

There were days like this for Alex and Charlie with their businesses; everything going into emergency drive, everything hurtling rapidly out of control, spiralling faster, only to be recovered in the nick of time. With Alex Davies especially, that was a story for Collage, anyway.

Charlie's private nightmare lay with vandals. He dreaded the day that some punk would walk into his shop and smash the place up, damaging the aquarium tanks and flooding the shop floor with tropical fish and water. Alex's private nightmare involved incompetent chefs. Will they order the right food in advance?" "Will they cook and prepare the meals within the 20 minute deadline?" And, "will that dastardly dog owner ever have his way and get Pépé into the restaurant?"

However, the purpose of Apollo 13 was a divine combination of personal nightmare combined with brainstorming combined with revelation. In that order, starring Alex and Charlie.

As you know, Charlie managed to persuade Alex of the need for Collage to acquire a tropical fish aquarium. He did so out of best interests really. Truly, as a friend and fellow entrepreneur, and more so as somebody who dined at Collage anyway, Charlie had an instant case in hand. Alex needed not too long to determine that his customers may appreciate the décor more with these fish, so a deal was struck up.

No problemo, except for the disaster. Delivery day lay ahead and Charlie had asked for Tim's assistance to deliver the tank to the restaurant. Word got out and Alex invited Ben to witness the experience. Ben just had to bring Pépé as well to keep him company. So there they were all four at Collage. Charlie pulled up in his Fish4U! van and Pépé began to get excited.

The back of the van was opened, Tim jumped in, Charlie grabbed the close end and out came the tank. As they walked into Collage, tank in hand, the dog wound his way around Charlie's leg and caused distraction. Ben called Pépé back again. He did come back, only via Charlie's other leg causing Charlie to lose his temper, his balance, and his grip on the tank. Smash!!! The water covered the Collage floor, the fish scattered in all corners of the restaurant and Alex howled with disapproval, "Man, that totally sucks!"

Alex, upon witnessing the scene of the wreckage on his restaurant floor, stared in abject terror for some moments. Then, being a sharp wit he commented that the floor needed a wash today anyway and rapidly proceeded to the kitchen to collect a bucket of water for the fish..... their time aboard was less than 90 seconds, so just maybe they would survive?

So, the brainstorming part. What to do with the fish. What to do with the broken glass tank and what to do with that danged dog? Shoddy workmanship? Or unaccountable interference? Ben felt and was held personally responsible for some time afterwards, so exercised his ethical brain about how best to deal with such a circumstance.

Alex collected the fish up in no time on a dustpan, and transferred them to the kitchen sink. He then swept the glass and mopped the floor. Charlie raged at Pépé. Ben stood in moral apologetic defence for his dog and a discount was worked out for the next tank which was delivered within the hour. Similar tank of fish, only this time no dog to interfere with the proceedings.

Alex gladly acquired a 25% price discount on account of the mess, and Charlie made note not to allow dogs in his own shop Fish4U!

This calamity was just one of several that occurred amongst these two. Alex was a quick thinker at the best of times, but on occasion that would lead him to lose his temper with a fool or half-wit. Some time went past since the incident with the dog and one day the unthinkable happened once again.

Collage was experiencing a fairly normal, quiet lunchtime and out of clear blue sky somebody walked into the restaurant for lunch.

"Hello man, sorry to bother you on this fine day, but I hear great things about your eatery here…"

"Yes, very well, please take a seat and we'll be with you shortly".

"Oh, well what I was going to ask, is I'm doing this bike ride from John O'Groats to Lands End and I'm raising funds for this incredible charity dude".

"Oh God, you mean you want me to sponsor you?"

"No, actually better than that…I intend to eat for free in every establishment I come across on my voyage en plein aire".

"You are kidding me? No way do we give to any old cobber. Especially not on Tuesdays. So you either pay for lunch or get out!"

"Dude that sucks, I want my free lunch! After all I have cycled all this way to 'Scar the borough' already. I deserve better treatment than that for sure! Please man, I'm hungry, I'm not carrying one penny".

"Tough titty 'dude'! Now if you'll excuse us we have business to conduct."

With that, the cyclist started to yell out loud "You suck, I rock, I'm the mean machine you get that, my legs are harder than your head man, I could eat here if I wanted but your establishment is just too bad. I wouldn't touch your spaghetti if it had sauce on it; I wouldn't swallow a profiterole even if it was fresh. I'm the man and if I say sponsored lunch that's what I get!"

With that outburst Alex picked up a chair and marched briskly towards this intruder. "That's it, call the paddy wagons, that's too far!"

He flung the chair into the cyclist's face and watched as his arms flew up to deflect the object. The cyclist grimaced with antagonistic delight.

"I'm the fit one – just you remember that one, fatty!"
"Fatty bum bum, fatty fatty bum bum," he began to sing out loud.

Alex raged at this point, he could take no more of this anti-Collage behaviour. He picked up the phone to the cops and told them to get there quick. Within one minute flat the cyclist had launched one last insult and high-tailed down the road still continuing a search for a sponsored lunch. Good luck man, gosh he must be hungry by now if that was his best attempt.

The police arrived after thirty minutes and played it all down saying that some punk had lost the plot. They never pursued any more of that nonsense. More important things to be doing.

Alex was a quick man, but when someone disrespected Collage like that he felt bad, real bad. He needed to chill out and speak to Melanie about the day's event, so handed the reins to Suzanna whilst he went upstairs to tell his wife about the day's nonsense. Suzanna could easily run Collage by now. She had much experience and gladly carried over that now once- again quiet lunchtime.

"Freaks will happen," they thought.
"Wonder what the incredible charity was? Maybe it was all total BS."
"Maybe he needs medical attention or something urgently?"
"He should have paid for lunch – no trouble with that – instead of which look what exactly he got – a chair in the face…..must have his wires crossed or something dumb like that".

Alex could have laughed, could have cried. Melanie just grimaced when she heard. She had heard worse before. From time to time these things will happen, she said. Nonethless Alex felt a prize rage about the fact.

Days turned into weeks, and weeks into months. Business as usual, subtle developments along the way, customers in, fed, watered, and out once again. Or in the case of Charlie, phone calls made, prospective clients contacted and aquaria delivered. The fact that Ben's dog had previously caused a disaster had washed over and their relationship was not affected.

In fact, Charlie had forecast an eventuality such as this. He figured that it would be part and parcel for running a small business – "you win some, you lose some, but make sure to sing when you're winning," in the words of Robbie Williams.

He left any singing and music-making to Claire, though, in reality. There was no complaining about this mode of happening. Alex was proud to have friends like Claire and Charlie. He was a proud man anyway, but these people really did it for him.

So what else could go wrong for them within their company? The list of the hypothetical was longer than the list of actual. So with that in mind, we should continue to focus on the actual, to home in on the 'what is', the 'way of it', the 'matter of fact'. Running an enterprise for these young men had become a major undertaking. Their lives were governed by the rules and regulations, the why's? and wherefores? But this did not prevent them from having a full life in other areas at the same time.

One day, an order came through from a hotel. They wanted some tropical fish in their lobby, in a tank. They were renovating and getting rid of a load of old interior designing. Meaning to replace it all with more modern décor, one step was to contact Fish4U! and elicit from Charlie what deals he would be happy to make for them on this quest.

He determined that a large tank to be located in a wall- mounting full of 7 varieties of 24 fish should do the job. He would be asking them for a fee of £185 for his services and recommended to come and install the tank within a two-week period, at a date and time to be arranged soon at their choosing. This would be the way of it for the Colombia Hotel.

The next few days were spent selecting the fish and transferring them into a large tank in anticipation of their delivery. The deal would include water filter, feed, cleaning apparatus, and a recommendation for whose Insurance to take up for the fish. Probably a standard Pet Insurance deal would cover the scenario.

Anyhow, a few days later, there was a phone call and they agreed to have the aquarium delivered the next morning between 10am-12pm. This was fine with Charlie. He arrived the next day promptly at 10am, and breezed into reception.

"Good morning, I am here from Fish4U!, here is my card, and the delivery is in my van outside."

"Ah, Mr Morris, pleased to see you. Thankyou for being so prompt this fine morning. Would you be requiring any assistance from our porter?"

"Actually, yes, that would be most appreciated. I couldn't manage the tank on my own as it is too large."

"If you would like to bear with us just two moments, I will give him a call on the intercom and then he will come at once."

"Oh, OK, thankyou very much".

Sure enough, two moments later the porter arrived on the scene.

"Mr Morris, pleased to meet you. The name's Malone; Stan Malone".

"Right then Stan, let's get cracking, shall we?"

"Yes, let's just."

The two men got to work and went out to the Vauxhall and collected the tank to bring inside the reception area. By this point the wall mountings had yet to be fitted, so Charlie returned to the van to collect the joinery tools and set to work on the fitting.

"Is there anything else I can help you with Mr Morris, or will that be all?" asked Stan.

"Well, once these fittings are in place I will need a hand placing the tank, please".

"Oh, alright, just give me a shout when you are ready".

Charlie got down to business and screwed, scraped, hammered, pencil-marked, and clattered for half an hour. Then he returned to the receptionist to call Mr Malone to help him with the tank.

"Right Stan, we need to get this aerator switched on as soon as possible to oxygenate the water. The fish need to breathe properly."

"OKey-dokey, you're the boss, just tell me when."

"Ready: one, two, three, lift."

And they lifted the tank of fish into place wriggling and writhing it. Then the aerator was plugged in by the socket and the water began to bubble gently.

"That should do the trick, now," said Charlie.

"Yes, it's a pleasure to be of service Mr Morris" replied Mr Malone.

The two men went their separate ways from that moment forth, never to meet again, and Charlie then wrote out an invoice and dropped it off at reception.

"Wish you well with the rest of your renovations, hope it all clicks into gear soon"

"Thankyou Mr Morris, thanks for coming, here's your cheque."

Then Charlie left the Colombia Hotel, got in his van, and returned to the shop some 2.5 km away.

The morning had been a coup and he rewarded himself with a cup of tea and called Claire, asking about her evening's arrangements.

She was chuffed about the hotel and they agreed to meet for dinner at Collage that night at 8pm.

It was a very relaxed, informal evening that night. Suzanna came to wait the table and asked how they were doing. They told her of the day's events and how everything appeared to be on track at the moment. Then she took their order. They both opted for a leek and potato soup starter, followed by chicken and chips for Charlie, and salmon with peas and potatoes for Claire. They shared a bottle of Australian Chardonnay as they dined that evening.

"Tell me Charlie…..what are we going to do if this whole thing falls through? What if nobody wants to buy any more fish? What if my records don't sell? What if…"

Charlie cut her off at that point: "Never mind the what if's! Let's just enjoy the what is! The way it is and looks set to continue."

"You are an optimist…that's what I like best about you – your attitude to life."

Charlie smiled displaying a set of strong, clean, white gnashers. He used Mcleans whitener twice a day (morning and night).

Claire sat looking at him curiously for a brief moment and then the soup came out which they both ravenously set to straight away after the day's exertions.

Suzanna wished them "Bon appetit!" as waitress then left them to return to the kitchen area for further instruction.

The restaurant was medium-full on this occasion. A gentle hum of sounds and clankings from all the occupants.

By the time they had eaten their main courses Alex had made his way out to talk with them. He wanted to thank Charlie for the aquarium in the restaurant. He said that some people had commented that it gave a 'nice, friendly touch' to the place. He just hoped that no further nuisance would come this way again all of a sudden.

He recommended the fruit salad for dessert and both concurred with this idea. Followed by a coffee and a chocolate mint. When they had finished their evening meal Claire suggested that they might go to a club for some dancing antics. The idea did nothing for him but he decided to humour her and they both made their way to Vivaz to see what was going on that night. As it turns out there were two bands performing that night and the music was uptempo.

Being in the mood for a jive they went straight for the crunch and immediately threw their jackets to the side and went to strut their funky stuff on the dance floor. Some people applauded this and had a laugh about the keen pair going for it. So long as they had the stamina and the legs, that would be all that counted.

They stayed there until two o'clock in the morning as it turned out, with alternative refreshment breaks and spells on the dance floor. They were exhausted by the time they got home and went straight to bed and slept solid until ten a.m. the next morning.

As it was still mid-week Charlie had to open the store Fish4U! He rolled out of bed and went for a shower and a coffee before lightly kissing Claire on her forehead and wishing her well for the day.

The business day was fairly standard with plenty of chores and odd-jobs to be on with around the shop. He made some phone calls to other stockists in the county and checked on prices and any interesting developments in the market. As he had internet connection in the back room of the shop Charlie was able to conduct some online research and send a few emails as usual.

Lunchtime came at 12.30pm and he went to buy a sandwich from the next door sandwich bar. He opted for ham salad with a bottle of pineapple Lilt and a jam doughnut, then returned to the shop to continue with the day's work. Claire phoned up to tell him about a new gig lineup that had been offered to Seachimp in Harrogate. A pub had offered them an evening slot in two months time, along with slots in York, Grimsby, Whitby, Hull, Beverley, and Skipton. So she was happy with all that.

They shared a moment's anticipation as the prospect of more touring became real. Maybe a bigger name would pick them up and give them a slot at some summer festivals? They both certainly hoped so.

The rest of the day was fairly eventless all in all, so Charlie went home and sat in front of the telly for a while that evening, watching a Lee Evans comedy show, and the News.

Some time went by and days became weeks became a month, and suddenly there were new orders to deliver and new songs to be sung. It was a happier time now. Both players had recovered from their previous ill-fated hang-ups and got on. So much so that to meet them you would never know by looking what life had been like only 18 months previously.

So, Apollo 13; what else could go wrong for Alex and Charlie?

This and that it would seem. Little things like smashed dishes, burnt food, rejected meals, payment problems, excessive noise makers in the building, other restaurateurs coming in to dispense advice to Alex when he was already perfectly competent to make his own decisions. Things like this seemed part and parcel for the business.

Then one day a bombshell. The business was his own small business (Collage for Alex, Fish4U! for Charlie). The tax man payed a visit. Boomph!!! Every year, an annual tax charge to be paid in full in order to keep running the business on the said premises. Ouch, what a stinger.

Pretty much all of the first year's profits had been invested in the store and then this. Charlie had to pay out for both the loans, and the tax man. This cut him right down to size. Like a Stanley knife working its way through a sheet of cardboard.

Alex had a slight advantage. He had been at it longer and had the ability to pay it in full within one month of receiving the bill. This kept him in business and the taxman happy. So a win-win situation all in all. All in the name of playing the game. Play it again, Sam.

And so it was, so it would be, so it always will be. Playing the game. Accepting the rough with the smooth, taking scoops from the quality box and levelling out the playing field with them. Swings and roundabouts, ups and downs, taking the see with the saw. Flights and submersions, helicopters and submarines. One minute it's coming in, the next it costs dear.

Anyway, that tax bill was quite possibly Charlie's biggest Apollo 13 moment. Alex could just deal with it, Charlie had to shake, rattle and roll for a while before he could actually adjust to the charge. He did it. He took the colossal, giant leap and dealt valiantly with the tax bill for the first time.

This would be an important lesson for him in working in the shop for himself, as entrepreneur-owner. He was far from alone in this ball-game. There would be many thousands of others wracked in the self-same problem. So he took comfort from this fact. He was never on his own anymore. Even his dad had begun to back him favourably with regards to his business. Previously he had no-goed, forestalled and twisted away from even the idea, but he had been coming round to the reality of it over the months and had begun to help in his own way.

Charlie was chuffed at that. A support network had begun to emerge. The receptacles were floating, the buoys were at work here in the harbour of greater business to come. The ships were afloat, the sailors on board, on deck, all hands at the ready.

Charlie could now thrive, he could play with the rest of them, fly the local territory, explore the terrain, although he wasn't one to rest on his laurels. He deserved the sanctitude that came his way whenever he found any.

Charlie was not a solitary figure. He had Claire, he had Alex, and he had his father. All these figures were adding up to support him throughout his venturing procedures. And venturing is exactly the ticket that he was striving towards.

Alex had had tough times. His ride had never been easy. Never one to sit on his haunches even when times grew hard, Alex had discretion, prudence, a sense of timing, he had integrity. Alex had a profound and instilled sense of what it was to be a successful human in the world of restauranting.

Alex could never grow distracted from the job at hand. He had an innate sense of concentration and focus. He could focus on making a slap-up gourmet nosh, or equally on screwing a screw into a wall-fitting or a piece of wood. He would always pay attention.

Adamantly, he refused to allow pets into the restaurant, but Ben was convinced that he would, one day, press the right buttons for Pépé to enter the premises. Whether there would be any purpose of dog accompanying master into Collage would remain to be seen, but there it was, Benjamin Williams taking on the might of Alex Davies.

"Dogs should wait outside, or better still at home," explained Alex to Ben one day.

"Yes, but he likes company…he's a very sociable dog you see," Ben replied.

"That's against company policy I'm afraid, Benbo. No animals allowed in Collage. It could ruin me!"

"Oh, that's nonsense - Pépé is a perfectly well-behaved Cocker Spaniel. The only nuisance he's capable of is yapping at the waiter," Ben continued.

"Even so, I'm sorry – no dogs in here. People would stare, people would complain when they tried to eat their dinner," Alex went on.

"Well, it's your loss at the end of the day" Ben said, "I'll be going where the dog goes and he with me. So you could be losing out on a customer if you're not careful".

"Are you getting arsey with me, Mr Williams? Please, spare me the time of day and take your gaping arse away from here before I shove a marrow where the sun don't shine," Alex attacked.

"Well, there's no need to be quite so hostile now. Very well, good day, Mr Davies. We'll meet again, no doubt?"

"Yes, indeed, good day Mr Williams. Until we meet again. Hasta la proxima," Alex concluded.

With that Ben walked away with Pépé, and Collage, once again, remained pet-free.

So there were quibbles and there was a bit of in-fighting amongst the crew members with regards to Collage and the dining, restaurant, business experience.

Tim too had a part to play in all this. He had continued training for quite some time over the months and continued to look towards the future meets that would inevitably take place. He had more association with Charlie than with Alex, probably to do with the fact that he had supported Claire through her darkest days.

Tim turned up at Fish4U! one day and went to speak to Charlie.

"Now then, fella," Tim greeted him with.

"Oh, hello there, Tim. How's tricks?" Charlie responded.

"Just calling in to see what's new really. Any troubles?"

"Nothing too great."

Charlie went on to explain to Tim about the tax man and the charge.

"Ouch, that must have stung you?"

"Yes, took me by surprise, actually. Anyway, a man's gotta do what a man's gotta do," Charlie explained.

They made a few jokes and Tim told Charlie about his training regimes and how the competition was currently looking. Suitably impressed, he offered him a delivery assistant job, but Tim turned it down in favour of sticking to his guns and continuing work at J Sainsbury's.

Life had begun to pick up a little over the months. Work was steady, early mornings, training in the evenings, and plenty to do along the way. All in all Tim was fully occupied and he, too, had a predisposition for making a line of activity and following it through to completion. He was a real stickler, a real attention-to-detail sort of guy.

The Apollo 13 with Tim had been and gone already. He broke his arm cycling in Dalby forest. What more could be said? The timing was poor, as his trials had been coming up fast. These were fast approaching and no longer merely idle conjecture, and Tim was actively looking to guard his place on Team GB. The triathlon was his life. Swimming, cycling and running. This is where Tim belonged, out on the course, on the track.

Charlie respected this very much. In a way, he wished that he could join him on the track, but in his heart of hearts his attention was purely on the store. He also respected the fact that Tim had caused no fuss when Claire had taken up with Charlie. Mainly because Tim had seen her through her worst moments from the perspective of a well-man.

It could have easily resulted in a conflict of interests had Tim been predisposed to anger easily. However, his interests were that of a platonic mentor. He was in no way, shape or form, one to despise, denigrate, deny, or otherwise cause damage to another human being. Especially somebody he had been fond of from an early age.

Charlie had won Claire as a girlfriend on the inside of a mauvaise predicament. They had found each other and colluded from that moment hence. Claire Halls and Charlie Morris had had their Apollo 13 moments already. The time had come to move forwards and strive unto new territory.

Tim had a valuable, valid, and valiant role to play in all this. He was an 'anointed' one, a select athlete with favourable attentions bestowed upon him. Maybe his time would come to shine big time? Only time would tell.

So here we had Alex Davies working Collage. Maybe, just maybe, an Apollo 13 for Alex would be The Flaming Squirrels cafeteria. He had decided to give it the go ahead. Suzanna Jeffries was in tow on this one. She had always expressed an interest in the business proposition. The opportunity to assist in running a café would occupy her every thought for quite some time to come.

'The Flaming Squirrels' was a brand new establishment in addition to Collage. For all those on board the proposition, well that would speak for itself, really. The main proponents were Alex and Suzanna. Of course, also with Melanie, his wife. She had given very careful consideration to the project as well. How would it affect the family environment? Would two small businesses be too much to bear thinking about?

Time would tell. And time did tell. The café opened up within a short space of time and Suzanna Jeffries was sworn in as Assistant Manager to Alex Davies' Ownership. How would it unfold? Well we hoped, as Collage had been thriving, so it seemed likely that an additional café could thrive, too.

Café culture seemed to be an esoteric thing. Not for everybody by all means, but comparing independent-branch coffee shops to the major chains would come into the equation in a big way for Suzanna Jeffries during her time here.

She had visited hundreds of cafes as a paying customer over the years just to get a feel for the different styles of enterprise. Her firm conclusion was that by far the most comfortable cafes were the independent-branch ones, where they actually got to know your name and made you feel at home.

She was delighted, over the moon in fact, to be on board The Flaming Squirrels café enterprise with Alex as gaffer. It meant the world to her. All her hopes and dreams had been pinned on running the show one day. In addition to physically running triathlons with her brother, she would now assist in running an enterprise 'show' in the cafeteria.

So again, an Apollo 13? Not so much this time, early days you see, too early for anything of that calibre to be occurring. So more like an Apollo 13 blueprint.

The design was set, their mission stated plain, and now the time had come to realise and operate two fully-functional hospitality units. All in the local vicinity. Would the people come? And if they did, would they be satisfied?

Time would tell, another day would unfold as sure as night follows day follows night follows day. As sure as the sun will shine, as sure as the rain will fall, time would decide the fate of The Flaming Squirrels.

Sounded a bit trite maybe, but no way, not on this earth, would Alex Davies back down from his ideas. He had the nous, he was experienced enough, and he had the staff to work for him when needed. The shifts would be covered. So what's new Barney McGrew? All sorts, you've only got to open your eyes and see the daylight, hear the birds sing, feel the breeze in your face, and whistle a jolly tune. That's what's new at the end of the day…whatever you made of it.

And at the beginning of the new day, immediately following the darkest and coldest of nights comes the daybreak. After the eleventh hour comes the refreshing sign of life. After Apollo 13 comes an overawing sense of satisfaction for a job well done; a calamity transformed into an achievement all at the hand of the maestro.

Apollo 13 comes and Apollo 13 goes for us all, but for Alex and Charlie they were at least equipped, equipped with the 21st century tools to run an enterprise. Collage would continue to make sense, Fish4U! would develop as best as possible over the months to come, and The Flaming Squirrels would begin to grow, just as an acorn turns into a giant oak, so would the businesses of Alex Davies become substantial in time.

Life was looking up for the crew, what once was down was now sailing through, and the reasons to live on had come in thick, fast, effusively; trials had become successes, traumas had been overcome and the Apollo 13 rocket was coming home to land.

Chapter 16
Team GB

Tim had won himself a place on Team GB as a triathlete. Aside from being an expert BMX bike rider, impressing the by-standers, Tim's skills were awesome. One minute he would be idling around engaging in some friendly banter, the next he would be on the ramps at the skate park. His style had become very natural, as though the BMX were an extension of his physical being.

How did Tim discover his penchant for BMX biking? As a kid, Tim first learnt to ride a bike, aged five. His father would push him along with and then without stabilisers at a progressive pace. As soon as the stabilisers came off Tim took off. Wheelies, bunny hops, endoes, 360s, jumps, bounces, whirls and twirls, all proceeded to join his fluid biking vocabulary.

Not surprisingly he had broken his left arm by the age of twelve, attempting new stunts. But not one to be perturbed, Tim grew up and on with his beloved BMX bike. His father was himself a cyclist – by recreation more than profession - but Tim had the full support of his dad. His mum found herself constantly concerning about more potential breakages. "Whino", Tim called his Mum in jest.

Anyway, Tim had risen through the ranks, and after countless star rides, tournaments, friendlies, amicable stunt park days, triathlons, and general BMX riff-raff encounters, he was on his way to London for the Summer Olympic Games 2012. For the second time, since Beijing 2008, BMX biking was to be featured as an Olympic sport. Not that Tim would ride a BMX there, as he was doing triathlon, but the prospect of this race intrigued him very much.

Tim's fitness was top notch (Shane and Suzanna could have vouched for that) after numerous triathlons together – Ripon, Scarborough, London, and Leeds-Bradford to name a few– his insurance company took a lot of persuading to accept him for a suitable accident and injury claim sheet.

His mastery of the BMX bike really became prominent at the age of 17. He had finished school after his GCSEs aged just 16 and joined the local J Sainsbury store as an assistant. After two years there, he had risen to become assistant manager and all his earnings would be directed into triathlon/BMX biking gear.

With an initial investment purchase of a £150 Univega and crash helmet, Tim's training really took hold after school was up at 16. Early mornings, later evenings, he knew his heart well enough to follow through with this one.

Of course, on proving his notorious skills several sponsorship offers came in for him – Diamondback, FreeAgent, Trek, Giant and Claud Butler – some merely a photo shoot, others actual equipment; all companies had reached a suitable level of being impressed to declare support and imminent backing for Tim Richardson (the *Star*).

The local bike magazines would feature Tim from the age of 15 pulling his stunts and racing, on the BMX bike. At the time he was the coolest kid in school. Fame and sponsorship formed from a very young age.

Tim, Shane and Suzanna had always been very much in this together. Their levels of ability clearly differed and occasional hostility or envious rivalry would distort their relationship temporarily. Their bond was mystical, magical, as though they had sworn a three-way blood oath on their competitive friendship. Maybe they had?

Tim was picked for Team GB Triathlon at the tender age of 21, a mere stripling, but damned convincing. While the other bikers knew Tim by looking, in his free time, the park would be his territory. Nobody ever would interfere when Tim took to the ramps. He would just love to blast out his heavy metal – rock music and pull off an array of impresario stunts for his buddies. Even his not-so-buddies could not help but be seriously impressed by this young rider.

Tim knew Shane from early pre-school days, and Suzanna subsequently came into his circle of friends as Shane's sister and fellow Triathlete. "What a bunch of antipodereans," Tim would utter to himself as he would pull off an incredible aerial 360 spin in front of the crowd.

He had reached a level where wiping out would not be an option anymore – but when it happened, he would know *how* to tumble on the ramps.

His BMX bike had taken him on incredible tours around the UK, and onto the Continent – France, Spain and Germany. He would meet all his biker friends and ride until ridden-out, all the while storing a fresh J Sainsbury's profile back home, making the money to self-support. This guy had it made. Now Tim's star was truly shining.

Tim rocketing to stardom had never been an easy ride, however. With his broken arm and nagging mother, his jealous comrades trying to tear him down (and succeeding from time to time), and public disorder fines for playing Nickelback, Evanescence or Muse at full whack, he certainly got a fair share of challenge.

Rattling, rolling, bone-shaking, volleying, skating, carousing, Tim could just do stuff.

The tedium of a day-job was relieved for Tim with a really welcome break of going to a solid training session. His best comrade on board a BMX would be Vinny, also a Team GB select since 2008, and what's more, Vinny was *for the cricket*. Being British, Vinny truly cared to keep a tally with the England cricket squad, and supported Yorkshire every summer season.

So, as far as Tim and Vinny were concerned, on board the BMX bikes they were warriors atop their trusty steeds on a mission. The mission was plain, the mission was clear – take their superb transferable skills and win in 2012. What could be clearer? Nothing they had ever heard of. Coaches, management, physiotherapists, advisers, sports masseurs, sponsors, bike maintenance staff, bank loans, all in. Everyone was in on the deal.

"Get Tim the Gold". Hell, he deserved it. "Take this boy to cycle heaven in London". "Let him rip the tits with Arnie"; "give him the space to fly high supremo". Tim had his calling-card so clear. Oh so fine, this young man on his bike. There would be time, of course, in future Games to occur if needed be. Tim the pioneer, Tim the king, Tim the man on two wheels.

And these two wheels were no ordinary two wheels. Take the Univega to the Diamondback and add a trick or twenty-three and you had the man. Tim the jive, Tim the rhythm, Tim the vibe – man on a bike. This God would live forever, forever young riding the bike. Tim would beat Mr Rip Van Winkle on the ride around the earth's belt. Tim would out-jump him as he idled along. Mr Winkle's beard grew too long and caught up in his chain mechanism. Tim flew through, clean shaven 'n all.

There never was any doubt about that contest. Mr Winkle dazed and confused, Mr Tim growing stronger, flying higher, riding harder, pulling the stunts, man, racing and pulling the stunts to make the difference, to make the place, to get on the team.

Tim had focus, such depth of focus. Nothing had yet caused distraction from this. No tits, no cock 'n bull, no derangements, no tittle-tattle could have denied Tim his place on the Team. Living the passion was his life, living the passion of his life. Tim was born on a bike. As he was born he flew out of mummy pedalling his trike down the corridor at two hundred miles an hour. The selectors snapped him up then and there. He was that good.

Born to impress, Tim the impresario. Vinny no less. Vinny could battle with Tim at the best of heights. How they would shimmy, duck and ride together. How the two collaborators would torment their souls for any day spent out of the saddle.

Taking Lance Armstrong as his chief source of inspiration, coming from pro-triathlon, Tim knew how to handle the bike.

Mike, on the selection committee, stumbled upon Tim at a continental meeting. Tim pulled off a particularly efficient series of "routine manoeuvres" to rapturous applause only to be greeted by a stranger introducing himself as 'Mike'.

Mike offered Tim a place on the Team and then subsequently came across Vinny within a very short space of time. "This BMX ride is a happening occurrence man. You bet!"

Next stop Sheffield, Glasgow, then Gateshead. The UK annual meets were due to come up sooner rather than later. Tim was well on track to pull in the points. What about J Sainsbury's? They were in on the act. Proving to be a quality investment, J Sainsbury's provided the meet refreshments for Tim and co and would do so for the above events.

Always reliable, mister Tim knew how to be a human angel as well as a star. He was unattached, no love yet, but an overwhelming, burning desire to come clean and do good at the London Olympics.

Being an Olympic virgin Tim would spend many an hour in meditation, pondering the why's and wherefores, not leaving too much room (if any at all) for the doubts, the what-ifs. No room for thoughts of failure. Tim had absolute certainty about his performance state. Tim had stepped-up. Tim was on the mark, ready to greet the world on his Diamondback ride. A stunning method employed by Tim…beat Vinny, "Vinny's for the cricket" – "I am for London - London calling."

What did Team GB *mean* to Tim? Pretty much everything available in a young athlete's dreams; lots of rocket-fuelled, action-packed moments. Top banana!

Tim was never one to give in all too easily, determining from a very young age to train harder, ride faster, stir crazier than ever before. His anticipation was at fever pitch. Bearing witness to the outstanding world tournaments since being a 4 foot whipper-snapper, Tim always was one to determine his winnings (or the odds at least) in advance. Born under the star sign Leo Tim certainly had the heart of a lion.

As for Vinny (Vincent as his dad called him to this day), his selection onto Team GB came from the North-East as well. That is another story though, born an Aries; so we will leave it at Tim and Vinny got selected to represent Team GB. Being realists – the glass neither half empty or half full – the glass of Tim and Vinny represented the opportunity simply to quench their thirst.

In this case, riding a BMX was neither safe nor dangerous, but represented the opportunity simply to flaunt the long-term skills built up from the foundation of a well-rehearsed youth.

Where was Tim's love-life I hear you scream? The truth was – Tim was on a one-track mission. No distractions, his love-machine was his velocipede. His fitness was one true desire. Nothing came between Tim and his training schedule. Nothing at all.

That is how he made it onto the Team. With a pure 110% dedication focused to the umpteenth degree. Tim's key equalled: focus.

Nobody would ever say that the lad got distracted for an hour or two, because he just couldn't afford to. His tactic? Constant And Never-Ending Improvement (CANI™). Ain't nobody who won't if you really look hard enough. Kaizen, Total Quality Management. Tim lived for this stuff on the paradigm of BMX bike-riding and triathlon.

Because for Tim life was in chunks. Blocks. Paradigms of existence. His favourite paradigm was of course riding the bike; however he had paradigms for friendships (Shane and Suzanna) and he had paradigms for leadership especially looking up to Ben as a mentor, and Alex Davies as an entrepreneur. His role at J Sainsbury's management fit this too. Mike, the selection agent played a key role here, too.

How did Tim fit into Plan 103f? Because he represented the ideal that Shane and Suzanna would never experience, selected for Team GB to ride out at the London Games 2012 in the Triathlon. On being on best terms with the lad, their best strategy was to support Tim. For sure, there be competitive envy, for sure there be a bit of tiffle-taffle. But their bond was solid as a rock. Plan 103f was for Tim the star lad. All his heart was in the riding, with J Sainsbury to fall back on if he were to fall through.

Plan A – ride at London, plan B – Win, plan C – make a packet at J Sainsbury – plan so on and so forth, until it got to the point where it would be just too darned depressing to even so much as contemplate what was to come next. And if all the above failed then we would have Plan 103f.

"Always look on the sunny side of the street", Tim had found the greener grass, nothing could be plainer. Personal motto "Win!" He was onto a winner here.

These were the ultimate words for Tim Richardson to hear that day. He knew from that moment onwards his career as a triathlete would reach a higher status than he had ever experienced before. It would not be a gift on a silver plate by any means. He would have to work at it, keep it, maintain his fitness and stay on top of the game. He wouldn't want to lose this.

His colleague Vinny was there on the BMX bike. They kept bumping into one another on the courses and at Team GB meetings. They always had a laugh together and got on and found the whole thing to be an absolute honour and privilege.

Well, time went past and the Olympics were fast approaching. Tim had been going through paroxysms of pre-event nerves despite his whole training and preparation. Shane always told him not to be so hung up about the outcome. There were so many world-class athletes going to be present at the event. He had secretly got thoughts that Tim would meet his match at the Games but continued to pep him up with enthusing comments whenever they were to meet.

His own fitness levels were astonishing, but never in a way to get to the highest class of Olympics or Commonwealth games. Shane was a 3rd degree blackbelt in Taewkwondo and an instructor. At an earlier age he had dreamed of getting to the Olympic Games. However, his moods and temper tantrums had him struck off the list by the officials and he would have to make do with the local clubs and regional area meetings.

Nothing wrong with that anyway. He was really delighted to be representing his sport as an instructor. He had read hundreds of books and magazines on the subject, trained hard and diligently for years on end and was reaping the rewards for his own fitness and elasticity.

His sister was impressed with him even though there were occasional arguments and disagreements between the two of them. Shane wanted to prove himself all the time and sometimes he would go off on one just for the sake of having his presence felt by those around him. He was glad that Tim had got into the Team and would therefore stand a chance at winning a medal for his country.

Shane had decided to travel to London to be there in person to show his support. Ironically it would mean travelling on the same train as Ben Williams – his pet hate – and Suzanna all at the same time. The Team travelled separately.

The time had come. It was the evening of the opening ceremony in London. Shane, Suzanna and Ben were sat in the stadium amongst 50,000 spectators. The teams all came out from countries around the world bearing their flags. Australia, Iceland, USA, China, France, Germany, Spain, Chile, South Africa, Nigeria, Samoa, Fiji, Cuba, UK, Japan, Ethiopia, Morocco, Kenya, Hungary, Poland, India, Pakistan, Russia, Georgia, and over two hundred more. The three looked hard and could just make out Tim and Vinny in amongst the Team GB select as they marched out into the stadium.

There was music and fireworks. The cauldron flame was lit and great announcements were proclaimed during the evening. Millions upon millions of people all around the world were watching the event on their televisions and on the internet. Everybody was cheering and applauding as the athletes paraded around the stadium in anticipation of the events to come, the adrenalin and potential medals awarded.

Shane yelled out "Way to go, Vinny, go get 'em tiger!"

Ben merely applauded, and Suzanna shouted "Bravo Tim!"

The opening ceremony seemed very exciting, full of pomp and hype and people coming from every direction. A day of unity for the people of the world. In spite of all the unrest and disturbances preceeding the event, here it was unfolding for all the world to witness. An Olympic spectacular, an extravaganza, an athletic bonanza on the face of all the world. One big family celebration!

The BMX biking was a relatively new sport for the Games since 2008 and Vinny was due to ride out and race very quickly on day eight of the events. Triathlon was due to occur on day 10. Tim would have to Swim 1.5km, cycle 40 km and then run 10km on his way to Olympic glory and national honour.

It was a tense time indeed. All the training, all the preparation, all the anticipation, all the advice and specialist skill accumulated over the years was being put to the test here in London.

So the three comrades had decided to see certain events during the three week period. Suzanna was keen to see the swimming, could Rebecca Adlington defend her titles? Ben wanted to witness the boxing, could James Degale do it again? and Shane had high hopes to view the Taekwondo tournaments, to see Aaron Cooke and Sarah Stevenson fight for a medal.

They were staying in a London hotel in separate rooms and kept in contact by means of mobile phone. Ben and Shane still didn't see eye to eye, but their contact time was minimal as they all wanted to do different things.

The two events where they would watch together would be the BMX ride and the triathlon. Other than this they were free agents. Shane made a bee-line for the sports centre and feasted his eyes on all the fit, flexible and agile martial artists. He was thoroughly impressed by what he saw and excited to be there, although it was a touch reminiscent of what he could have been in another life. Shane was incognito within the arena and glad of it.

Suzanna headed straight for the 50 metre swimming pool and spent the entire week supporting the swimmers. Her favourite event was the individual medley. Butterfly, backstroke, breaststroke and then freestyle. Would Michael Phelps be back? She screamed her guts out for the British swimmers.

Ben felt a fighter at heart when he managed to wangle his way to watch the boxing tournament in progress. No bets placed however, his ethics got in the way of this. He was thrilled when James Degale stepped into the ring to defend his title.

The three walked around the Olympic Village with the two stars Tim and Vinny. Although not for long, as they were both too focused on their events to come. Vinny especially was excited and totally pumped up to be there. He mentioned about the rowing and the sailing. Tim talked a little about the Modern Pentathlon.

Anyhow, the eighth day arrived and Vinny was due to perform on his BMX bike, the second time ever for this discipline. The crowd was full of youths into the cycling scene so they would be hard to please. The judges were not going to be light-handed. So Vinny went out and gave it his heart and soul. The heat was on.

The race was on, he made a dozen rapid rides through the heats and landed smoothly in the final round of the show. Down the slope, over the ramps, round the bends and totally launching into a high jump and a handstand out of the saddle, he was in fine form today. Tim was impressed. He knew what it was like.

Vinny made a thorough performance and the home crowd fans went wild. He waved a salutation to everyone and of the 12 finalists, only two guys had a serious tumble. Nothing broken, but a medal chance gone up in smoke.

Shane laughed at this misfortune. It looked spectacular as it happened. All in the nature of the sport he speculated.

The moment of truth. Would Vinny win a medal for Team GB. As it happened, the Gold went to Latvia, Silver to USA, and Bronze to France. "Oh man, that just sucks ass!" Tim hollered. He was a bit concerned for his colleague as they had such a strong bond there between them. He knew from this what a strong field of competition lay ahead. He would have to spend the next five days very carefully indeed in final preparation. The five of them met after and went for some pasta to eat. Vinny was disappointed. He knew he had given it his all. There were no improvemements he could have made to the performance. The judges had downgraded the

English purely out of the others' graceful presentations. The show was a real spectacle.

They munched their pasta with little to say. Nobody wanted to say the wrong words at this time. Vinny left them to go and watch the rowing event and cool down. His dream had been shattered, but at least he got to be there. He was still an Olympic athlete after all.

Days went by. There was sailing, equestrianism, athletics, weight-lifting, tennis, boxing, gymnastics, badminton, table tennis, taekwondo, fencing, archery, wrestling, shooting, and so many other disciplines going ahead. Medals were being won right, left and centre. Day ten had finally come round.

Tim was on the line. Shane, Ben, Suzanna and Vinny had positioned themselves at four different points along the final running stretch. They would cheer him on as he came running home ahead of the game.

Tim heard the starting pistol and made a quick dive into the water. He remained amongst the front few during the swim. He received kicks to his chest on several occasions, almost swallowing some water in the process. But he battled on like a true warrior.

By the time they had got out of the water he was in fifth position after 1.5km. A 200 metre dash to the bicycle transition. Off with the swimwear, on with the cycling shoes and off he went on his wonderful Trek Madone 4.0, the self-same model that Lance Armstrong won a famous Tour de France on one year.

He was off with 40 km to go. A battle to keep his position lay ahead. Mr Tim Richardson riding strong, Mr Tim Richardson had trained for long, Mr Tim Richardson about to beat the throng.

The cycle ride took his breath away. Many national symbols and sights passed by as they all made their way round the route. Tim was breathing hard and by the halfway mark had lost three positions. He was now in eigth position with another 20km to go. He decided to pull out all the stops and reach for that other level which lay beneath his conscious realms.

He hoisted his mainsails and caught a good wind making steady ground. By the 30km marker he was in 4th place and once again in with a fighting chance of gaining a medal. They arrived at the final transition at the end of the bike ride. Tim hopped off his Trek Madone 4.0 and hurriedly put on his Asics air Nimbus trainers. They were sponsored trainers and he had rated them highly so was glad to use them in his race.

With 10km to go, there was no time to lose. A mad rush for the finish line thus ensued. Tim was in no mood to let anyone else take his title. He had stepped up. He was going for it and nobody would stand in his way to get that position and a medal for Team GB. He was a panther, a leopard, a cheetah, he had the fleetest feet on the planet. The wind was blowing him along like a ship in fine sail.

He probably did hear Ben as he passed by at the 5km marker, he must have heard Suzanna as he stormed the 7.5km point, he may have even heard Shane as he came round the 8km corner, but the only voice he could really hear was his inner voice telling him to go for it, to reach for the stars, and beat those other goons who were running as well.

He ran like the wind and had a sprint finish in the home straight. Building on all he had ever known, done, trained for and achieved, he was flat out. No previous result would be as big as this, he had to win. Busting his gut wouldn't matter, digging deeper into his soul for those ultimate reserves would never be a problem. Tim was flying, he had to win now. All he had ever lived for was here and now. History in the making. Reaching out, stepping up, if Phelps could do it 8 times at one Games then Richardson could at least make 1 title. He had to. He did! Tim Richardson sneaked a victory on the line. The sprint finish proved in his favour. Fate had handed him the title.

An exhilarating performance for all the world to witness. He collapsed momentarily in emotional exuberance. The first familiar voice he heard was Mike the agent in the endpoint. He thoroughly congratulated Tim and then Vinny came over to say a few words.

"Wheeeewe! That was some performance dude. You rocked, you got the Gold medal. The whole world saw you, you're a star, a top banana man," said Vinny.

"Yeah, I'm a bit puffed at the moment mate, that American was a close shave and almost just too good. I never knew he could move like that – until now!" replied Tim.

"Mm-mmmmm," Vinny mouthed.

They walked to the changing area, and by this time Shane, Ben and Suzanna had made it to the area and were asking Vinny for the final result. As soon as they heard they cheered, and Suzanna made to hug Tim. He was glad of the support. Even though he was too focused at the time to acknowledge them as he passed by, he was delighted they had been there.

Now they were all back together again, they had to make their way to the Podium stand for Tim to collect his medal. He did so with grace and dignity, shaking hands with the USA Silver triathlete, and the Portuguese Bronze, then receiving a peck on his cheeks from the gorgeous female presenter. He had won the Gold medal for Team GB and the UK and now his games were over. They would be forced to look ahead to the future and make new plans for further events.

So the Team GB buddies, Tim Richardson and Vinny 'for the cricket' had played their part in the London Games 2012. They were fit young things. Prepared and ready, but on the day the Olympic Gold went to the better man, and that was Tim Richardson.

They spent the remainder of the week in London to look around as tourists before catching the train back up north, home. Vinny returned to Newcastle in the team bus and Tim to Scarborough. Shane, Ben and Suzanna were now seeing more eye-to-eye as a result of their experiences in London. The trip was a once in a lifetime opportunity and meant more to them than words could ever say.

Tim had a few comments from strangers who had seen him on the telly. He had post waiting for him at home and was delighted to find some more sponsorship offers in line. Also, a TV show had asked him to come and be interviewed about the triathlon race he had just had.

He would be glad to accept on both occasions.

And so life was to go on, and Tim would have to wait another four years before attempting for the second time, to defend his title and win another Gold medal. Anything was possible, he was young. He figured that if Sir Steve Redgrave could win Gold five times on the trot, Matthew Pinsent four, Michael Phelps eight, Usain Bolt three world record Golds, then at least he should keep trying and keep his pecker up. There was hope to be had, he should stick to the game plan and step up the training, get better coaching, focus harder, and learn from further competitions.

There were still the Commonwealth titles in the meantime to be stabbed at. He had fresh thoughts, youthful aspirations, and the skills with the means to get there. Tim Richardson was born again – anew, renewed, refreshed and ready for the next day. A 2nd place result would not grind him down. It was his first attempt and he was ready for the next.

Mike from the selection committee had explicitly told him to look ahead once again to 2016. A home crowd and a native medallist made the world of difference to his esteem. A morale-booster if ever there was one.

So back to family. Not just family, but a very proud family. His commitment had paid off. J Sainsbury's were willing to keep him on the staff if he wished, although now he had made it this far with the athletics, time would be hard pressed. He had to make an important decision.…."do I stay here and continue training, or would that extra time make that bit of extra difference?"

He thought it through and talked to Ben, his mentor about the matter. "The training could be crucial," Ben told him straight. "That extra mile might be just this," he continued. "If you keep working at Sainsburys you may never know anything different. You're a star now Tim, think about that, why don't you?"

Tim thought for a moment and replied, "I don't want to just walk away from a long-term job. I've been doing this thing for years now since I left school. It would be like stabbing them in the back or something".

"They even sponsored all my training so far," he continued.

Ben took a turn to think for a while. Then he came up with an idea: "Why don't you stick at it for another six months with the new training regime. After that time, decide for definite what it means to you in the view of London. Speak to your boss and see what they come up with. Personally I would seriously think about moving on now. Changes happen, you've come on such a long way already in such a short space of time."

Tim nodded wisely. He liked what Ben was telling him but found it hard to accept immediately that he would have to leave his job and all the people behind with whom he had been working for all those years. A new lifestyle lay ahead for him and he would have to quickly grow accustomed to this fact. Hard though it was, he had been an amateur athlete and now the pointers were for him to go pro.

This was a whole new ball game, with a whole world of different connotations to it. A scary thought, even though he was not intimidated easily.

As for Vinny, he would stick to his BMX biking in the North East. 'Radical skater magazines' had gone wild for him to model for them. New clothes, bikes and gear had come in in droves and Vinny was favoured as the North East's BMX Olympian. He even got a mention at the Yorkshire cricket club with his photograph in the bar.

There was a gap of many months before Tim and Vinny heard from each other again. Ben had grown closer to Shane now and their differences were seemingly overcome. Suzanna was in the picture as well. She still admired Tim very much, but the proximity to Ben over the last year or two had meant that they were getting on better than ever before. They had embraced and kissed whilst in London, and everything was still cool after that.

Tim was the star, no kidding. He had an interview with Tim Don, the senior men's World Champion triathlete. The interview was on BBC radio 2 as part of a sport's awareness programme, hoping to reach out to other fans and wannabe's. It worked. There were phone calls and fan mail for the next few weeks. He was living a different life already.

Ben had a personal hero as well. Whilst he had watched the boxing contest he had been thinking of James Degale. He had seen him on telly at Beijing 2008. Ben was more philosopher than fighter, but the spirit lay in the same profound field. Amir Khan had also made a massive impression on his psyche at Athens 2004.

Suzanna used to watch the sailing as a kid. When Ben Ainslie started to win all the medals in 21st century Games, that had left her as pleased as punch. She was impressed by the versatility of the sailors. The sailing team at Beijing had won more medals and performed the best that a GB sailing team had ever achieved.

Shane still secretly hankered after his own place on Team GB. This would never come. He knew it really, but the thought ticked away at the back of his mind. He had his own rules and his family were keen for him to stick to the science lab rather than getting caught up in the impossible. He could do some mean tricks in a Physics lab. He was known for causing electrocutions in certain cases.

Meanwhile back home Claire and Charlie had been huddled around the TV set watching every move in those far away places. They were really chuffed that Tim had done justice to his talents; momentarily dreaming of their own results, but delighted.

Alex had made a welcome reception for the returning hero one night in Collage. There they were, the 'crew' plus a few others all gathered to celebrate the latest achievement. There was singing and dancing and people dressed up in their finest garb to commemorate the star.

Scarborough was ablaze with wonder. Jonathon Bateman came to personally congratulate Tim and to warn him that he would be on the track in future Games. They grinned warmly and understood that this was a challenge for both of them.

So the summer of 2012 closed with good times, and on into the autumn. "What a difference a day makes and what a difference with you," sang Ben to Suzanna as they left that night. She brushed it off as inane. They were singing within anyhow. Claire even wrote a verse to the star:

> Tim, you're a star
> You've run so fast and so far
> Were it not for you
> We may never have pulled through
> So I thankyou for all your heart.
>
> You made it to London
> Although not always fun
> More than words can say
> You really saved the day
> You and the Olympic rings.
>
> For us all you came in first
> Of this you long had sure thirst
> You are a force to be reckoned
> That London Gold really beckoned
> It's no mystery – you're in history
>
> Triathlon can be very long
> Especially to beat the throng
> Driving in a car
> Would not seem so far
> You're no beginner – you're the winner!
>
> Tim you're a star
> You've run so fast and so far
> We're all proud
> To say it out loud
> From Penzance to the Grampians
> You are in with the champions!

Chapter 17
Pépé 2

The years rolled by and Pépé had grown into a full sized dog by now. Ben had trained him well all that time and seen to it that he had been nurtured through and through. Pépé had come to recognise him as his master and was very loyal indeed. A pleasant tempered animal, barking only occasionally at other dogs in the street, or at strangers passing by the house on an evening whilst looking out of the kitchen window.

Ben had dramatically grown in confidence in this period of time, having experienced three major breakthroughs in his life and work. It all began when Pépé was still a puppy dog and his master had just been granted a position at the Scarborough campus as an ethics professor. Ben had, up until that time, been single for many years and read so much that he had become something of a guru, an oracle who attracted the respect and intellectual attention of many young students who he had had the privilege to teach.

Since joining forces with Tim at the triathlon, and witnessing him win the Gold medal at the London Games, Ben's relationship with Suzanna had really begun to blossom into something worthwhile. Whereas once there would have been animosity and a sense of void there was now more a sense of togetherness between them. Even Shane had begun to accept that they were a good match.

Ben could be strict at times, a disciplinarian, a stern demeanour could come over him at any given time thus affecting his disposition towards others. This didn't matter to her though. She saw his true self, the man within – behind the blinkers of a surface visual.

He could be profound at times in many ways, and in conversation this would become apparent. Not one to follow the charts or the football every week, more one for the classics and a pipe to smoke with a quality newspaper. He liked to read an unbiased paper so tended to go for the Independent during the week and the Guardian at the weekend.

A heavy read to be sure. Unimpressed with the Sun or the Daily Star he liked to be informed about what was going on in the world. An educated specimen, he knew a thing or two.

On a Wednesday afternoon Ben would visit the local pet store and buy some special treats for Pépé. Ranging from gnawing bones to choco doggy drops, there would be something new every week for him. He fed the dog half a jumbo sausage and biscuits with water every day for lunch often preceded by an hours walkabouts either in the park or on the beach.

Weekends would be a day trip in the car along the coast to Filey or Bridlington, maybe north to Robin Hood's Bay, Whitby or Saltburn. Ben would eat fish and chips whilst Pépé would have to make do with dog biscuits.

These expeditions went either accompanied or alone. Sometimes Suzanna would insist on going along as well for a walk. On occasion Ben would invite Tim out for a leg-stretch; schedule depending. They still had a mentor–student relationship going on there, but Tim had a new destiny now so was increasingly moving on towards a new crowd, including the prospect of gaining a different coach to work with.

Suzanna liked to talk about fashion to him for some reason. So often the big names would crop up in conversation: Calvin Klein, Marco Polo, Gianni Versace, Yves St Laurent, Ralph Lauren, Gucci, Christian Dior, Prada, John Galliano, and so on. She liked to go clothes-shopping from time to time, so knew what to look for in terms of cut, colour, texture and design aesthetics.

Ben would tend to just listen as he was filled in with all the details. There was a lot to be learnt in this manner, by just listening to others. The material was good quality and interesting to listen to. He was glad to know about these 21st Century clothes from a first hand experience.

Pépé would walk alongside them wagging his tail and sniffing for sticks and scents in the pathway and undergrowth. Life was looking good for Ben now.

Jamie Kershaw

Upon return home after their jaunts in the countryside and coastal areas he would set to reading some works of literature and pull out a pencil marking any inaccuracies or inconsistencies in the material. This would occupy much of the evening time schedule.

Ben lived just off Falsgrave Road at the top end of town so there would be noise as traffic passed by in the street, and pedestrians talking away or singing or shouting as well. He was happy with the life that he was leading. A fairly average chap on the whole, with assets that made it all seem worthwhile. He had plans and he had had results along the way. He was OK where he was and determined to stick at it.

He had a big idea to win the lottery and played on a Saturday evening every week. Generally speaking, he would be at home to watch the show on television and check his ticket against the results as the balls rolled down the chute.

Much of the time there was nothing doing. Occasionally he would win £10 from three numbers coming up. His lucky numbers were the same every week plus one line of lucky dip. He played 7, 10, 13, 27, 36, 45 as his set of 'sure-to-win' balls. He felt confident that one fine day they would come up – all six – and he would walk away with a healthy sum to his name. Having played already for over seven years the odds were increasingly in his favour.

If he ever missed the Saturday night show there was always the online lottery website to check up on. He had heard about the European lotteries in France, Spain and Germany but never got round to playing these games of chance. Just the National Lottery at home in the UK. He had come up with the reasons.

Somebody once told him, "Ben, you know that women are like playing the lottery; you should never give up just because you don't win the first time!" He had taken that to heart and taken it as his cue to keep playing, keep trying, and keep high hopes along the way.

Now that he had in effect won a girlfriend, he wanted to make the transition from mediocre to highly affluent, wealthy and prosperous. In his heart of hearts he desired success. This would be something that would come for him, he figured.

Suzanna knew about his regular flutter and sometimes jibed about it. She laughed that if he won she would be swept off her feet into the life of a millionaire professor. A rare combination indeed. They had their hopes and dreams together anyway.

It got to that time on Saturday evening and they were in together watching the box as usual. The show was in progress. Ben had even answered a lot of the quiz questions correctly (with her assistance). They laughed that he ought to go on the show one time and see how he would get on with it. At this point in time it seemed to be something for the future years, rather than an instant leap for it.

The numbers came out: 11 (no), 22(no), 31 (no) 36 (yes), 44 (no), 45 (yes). Just two numbers had come up out of the six. So, nothing doing yet again. He would have to wait another week to get rich. They spent approximately ten seconds in dismay, then scrumpled up the ticket and got on with the evening at hand.

They prepared some hot crumpets with golden syrup and a pot of tea, then continued watching TV together for a while. A documentary about African wildlife was showing for the next hour so they turned their attentions to this show and indulged in their snack.

Pépé was mooching around the living room, chewing the sofa legs and making funny slobbery noises, alternately lying on his back and rolling round asking for his tummy to be tickled. This was obliged for a moment whilst watching the TV show.

Round about 11pm it was time to go to bed for the night. They were staying in tonight so Ben stretched his arms above his head and yawned out loud. He asked, "Would you like to stay over tonight or would you rather get back home?"

Suzanna said that she would rather not walk alone at this time of night, so would it be alright if she stayed over?

Ben told her that 'of course that would be fine. The spare room is made up already. What time would you like to get up in the morning?

"Oh, Sunday morning, I might go to church tomorrow at 11am so anytime around 8-9am would be fine."

With that she went up to the room and closed the door and that was the last Ben saw of her that night. He was fine about that arrangement and sent Pépé to bed in his basket before switching off all the lights and brushing his teeth. He got to bed at 11.30pm that night.

He put his head down and went out like a light. Then around 1.30am he was woken up by the sound of Pépé barking wildly. He wondered what was going on so slipped his dressing gown on and bravely went down the stairs to see what all the fuss was about. All of a sudden he saw an apparition in the kitchen, a clatter, a bang of pots and the back door was hurried open and the intruder ran out into the night jumping over the fence into the back street. Pépé had scared him away. All that noise had done the trick.

How he had got into the house was another question. On closer examination Ben saw the key was still in the door. He had forgotten to lock the door in his haste to get to bed. A haphazard mistake to make.

The first instinct he had was to rush up to Suzanna's room and see if she was OK. Then he decided to scrutinise the scene and determine what, if anything, had been stolen – and wondered why had he been targeted. Pépé had been an absolute hero. He had scared the burglar before he had chance to cause any real damage.

As it happened, Suzanna poked her head around the door and asked what was going on. They decided that nothing valuable had been stolen, but she insisted that they call the police and state their case of trespassing.

"There has just been a break-in and attempted burglary."
"Where are you calling from?"
"Falsgrave Road".
"What's your name?"
"My name is Benjamin Williams. My dog scared him away!"
"We could come over right away for a statement if you want?"
"Maybe in the morning would be best. I forgot to lock my door."

"That would be careless sir, wouldn't it."

"Was anything stolen?"

"As yet, it looks like he just ran for it."

"Did you get an identity at all?"

"Just a shadow – about 5'10'', with a beanie hat on and dark jumper."

"OK, we'll send someone to patrol the area. See you in the morning."

The call ended and Ben locked the door then they all went back to bed feeling a little disturbed by the experience.

In the morning they were up and breakfasting by 8.30am. There was a knock on the door, and an officer presented himself to them. The inquiry lasted not too long in all and then he left with the case in hand.

By 10.45am they had dressed up smartly and were on the way to the local church, an evangelical centre with a band playing Christian rock music. Pépé was given the run of the living room in the meantime. Unbeknown to him he was the talk of the morning in the church. A super-dog if ever there was one.

Ben and Suzanna shared their story with some others and were gratified to receive some compassionate understanding. They were actually still in a state of mild shock that somebody would actually get into their house after hours at all. Ben was told off for being so careless as to leave the back door unlocked. A communal prayer went around for Ben, Suzanna and better times to come. Thank God for the dog.

Nothing had actually been stolen and Ben was glad that the lottery ticket had not actually been a winner that time. Had it been so, the burglar's finding it would have been a disaster. He had only ever won the minimum prize so there was still plenty of time for improvement in this area.

The other church-goers eventually filed out and Ben returned home with Suzanna. She was relieved that Pépé was alright and no harm had been done except for a few disturbed implements in the kitchen that night. She feared that the intruder would return, so told Ben to install a double bolt on the top and bottom of the door, making entrance impossible from the outside.

The event had caused Ben to reevaluate the safety of living on Falsgrave Road. Why had he been targeted yet nothing stolen? What did they want? For what purpose did the trespasser break in, in the first place? Was it for a document? Some money, valuables or the DVD player? What an enigma he thought.

Nothing was lost, just a bit of sleep and a knock to his sense of dignity. They put on a brave face and got over the event and got on with their day. Pépé was glad to see them when they returned home once again. He yelped and jumped up to Ben's chest as he entered the living room.

They decided to make a Sunday lunch, feed Pépé and then go for an afternoon stroll to digest their meal. Suzanna prepared the vegetables – the roast potatoes, mash, carrots, sprouts and parsnips – whilst Ben dealt with the roast beef and gravy. They had a fruits of the forest cheesecake for dessert, and Pépé ate his usual sausage and biscuits, although he was given extra biscuits for being so brave the night before, and Ben decided to give him the bone from the joint as well after being carved.

They were content with that and sat for a few moments deciding where to walk. They agreed to head to Peasholm park, North Bay, round the headland, South Bay to the spa, up the coastal footpath and back home along the roadside once again. The weather was fair, with the sun shining in between clouds, and a gentle breeze – not too hot and not too windy, so ideal for a Sunday stroll.

Pépé enthused as his lead was brought out for walkies. He knew what that meant….an outdoor adventure in the big, wide world. There was nothing that he liked more than an afternoon walk with Ben and Suzanna.

They set off and walked towards the park, when of all the surprises they bumped into Claire and Charlie enjoying some Sunday sun by the lakeside.

"Hello there," Ben said to Charlie.

"Hi Ben," came the reply.
Suzanna and Claire smiled at one another briefly.

"Fancy meeting you here," Charlie declared.
"Yes, what a coincidence," Ben responded.

They talked for a moment about the night's events and told them how Pépé had heroically scared away the intruder. Claire raised her eyebrows and looked alarmed for a moment.

"But he went, right? And the dog scared him? Gosh, that's not what you would need at one o'clock in the morning!" she said.

Neither couple wanted to join the other for the afternoon, so they continued on their way and walked Pépé onwards round the North Bay promenade. There were many other pedestrians walking along, and vehicles passing on the road on this occasion, like a typical Sunday afternoon by the North Sea.

Ben suddenly reflected that Charlie had seemed a bit distant in the park, as though at arm's length. He criticised himself for being so personal, though. In his heart of hearts he was glad to have met them and would not want to be thought of as a backstabber, so enjoyed his current company and the walk at hand.

When they got to South Bay, the amusement arcades were packed full of kids and teenagers, the marina was full of boats of all shapes and sizes, and the cafes that were open had many people sitting outside in the pavement seating area drinking and communicating together about this, that and the other.

Ben preferred the tranquillity of North Bay to South Bay, which was more touristy and full of tack. Although it was only South Bay that offered donkey rides for the kids and it was only North Bay where you could find surfers catching some waves when the tide was right.

They walked on, letting Pépé off the lead on the beach to play ball and be free for a while. As they arrived at the Spa Ben speculated that maybe Seachimp would one day perform there amongst others. He had been to a number of concerts in this venue, including the September jazz festival in previous years. There were some

263

incredible artists playing, ranging from Courtney Pine, Stan Tracey, and Clare Teale to Barbara Dickson. He appreciated music although never able to play an instrument himself.

Suzanna was keen to attend a concert with Ben, so made mention that it would be a good idea to go sometime soon. They walked up the steps and Ben nearly tripped, partially twisting his ankle as they climbed. Fortunately it was not painful for longer than five minutes so they resumed their walk and headed for the coastal footpath.

Once they had climbed this then Scarborough looked altogether distant from here. With the distant castle on the headland hilltop and the harbour down below, the sight was altogether rewarding for their exertions.

Later that afternoon they returned home feeling exhausted from the walk so put up their feet and flicked on the – guess what- television. There was nothing of interest on, so Ben decided to do some work and mark some of his students' papers. Suzanna decided to go back to her family home and thanked Ben very much for the weekend's excitement. She said 'Goodbye' to Pépé and then left the building.

So, once again, it was Ben and Pépé guarding the fort. Pépé roamed around chewing objects, assorted items and affects unbeknown to Ben, who was hard at work in the study room. This went on for four hours before he looked up for a break. Pépé had managed to slobber all over the chair legs, and chewed up a cushion too. It was mangled and in a state of doggy disrepair, so Ben scolded him - and then proceeded to pat him on the head in forgiveness. It wasn't that big a deal, after all he had saved the day.

The weeks went by and Ben still hadn't won the lottery. Every Saturday evening he would check his ticket numbers, and every Saturday evening the same disappointment would come. One number, maybe two, maybe even three on occasion. Ben would joke with the bar staff on campus to put the bill on his tab – he would pay it when his winning ticket came.

This was only in jest, however, and they knew full well that he would pay for his drinks, regardless of being staff. There were certain staff privileges but that did not extend to free drinks in the canteen. He would have to pay, the same as anyone else.

Then it came. Ben was at home as usual doing his work, but he had become so absorbed that he forgot to switch on the show. At 10 o'clock pm he looked up. Pépé was in the room laying down relaxed. He suddenly remembered to switch on the teletext to check his numbers. Page 555 BBC One; 'Let's have a look then, shall we Pépé?' he said to the dog.

"Ok, what have we got this time?" Ben said.
"08, 22, 24, 37, 38, 49".
"Hmmmm.....oh....oh my goodness, yikes, wow, blimey, Pépé we've matched five on the lucky dip," Ben yelled excitedly. "We got the lucky dip – we got five" he yelled. "Quick man, double check, just to make sure – no, this can't be - maybe it is another week's numbers, or Daily Play, or Thunderball?"

"Hang about – we've got the bonus ball too!"

Ben went through the numbers for a second time...."08 yes, 22 yes, 24 yes, 37 nope, 38 yes, 49 yes! Yes! Yes! Yes!" he became excited all of a sudden. "Pépé we're in the money! The bonus ball is 37. Now just how much exactly do we get for this?"

Ben, at first, was lost for words. He wasn't sure whether to call Camelot or whether to call Suzanna. He decided to call her first to share the news.

"Suze, hi it's me Ben....."
"....yes, yes fine thankyou!"
"Now I have something to tell you here – "
"- Suzanna, I think we just got five numbers and the bonus ball on tonight's lottery.....Yes, it's the truth; no I'm not joking! ....Can you check for me please? No, not the usual – it's the lucky dip".

Ben went on for a moment and then gave her the two lines of numbers that he had just played. There was a silence for two and a half minutes whilst she went to check. Then all of a sudden she said:

"Ben, my God, we've done it – just one number away from the jackpot – it must be at least £100,000 – one hundred big ones, one hundred G's – what are you gonna do?" she asked.

Pépé could sense that something was up, something going on, and he began to bark with curiosity. "Hey Pépé, calmez-vous, we've only won some dough," Ben told him. "Woof, woof," said Pépé once again.

"You should phone Camelot instantly," Suzanna instructed. "Get back to me afterwards, and let me know the score," she ordered.

"Right then," Ben replied, "back soon."

With that he hung up and clenched his fists in victory, yelling "Yes!" Pépé responded with a doggy "yes!" and then he called the magic number on the back of the ticket to Camelot.

"Good evening."
"Good evening Sir, Camelot here, what can we do for you?"
"I believe that I have five numbers and the bonus from tonight's play."
"Right then, let's have your numbers, Sir, and we will confirm for you."
"OK," said Ben, "Here goes…08, 22, 24, 37, 38, 49"
"Well, well, well – congratulations indeed Sir – that is indeed a five number and bonus ball match. What is your name, and where do you live?" they asked him.
"My name is Benjamin Williams, and I come from Scarborough in North Yorkshire".
"Right Ben, the procedure is as follows – we will send out a couple of representatives to you with the cheque, a bottle of champagne, and a camera. The cheque for you will be…….drum roll……£187,500 – this prize is the same for three lucky people tonight - all we need to do is arrange a date and time and you may bring your friends and family to the party."
"That's great" said Ben "I can't quite believe it, but that is just brilliant!"
"Well, Ben – congratulations once again and see you soon".

The call ended and Ben felt elated. He was 32 years old and now had some money in his life. That was more than five year's wages in one fell swoop, tax free. He had never before won a major prize. He wanted to call Tim and the crew, but remembered to call Suzanna first of all.

"Suze – it's £187,500 – yes God's honest truth – cross my heart and hope to die – they will come to Scarborough on Wednesday with the cheque".

She let out a whoop of exultation as the reality kicked in. A real prize, though not millions or the jackpot, it was a real coup to have this happen all of a sudden. Ben had been an average guy, a lecturer at college, a singleton, a little eccentric, a little bit of a leader with Tim, and now a cash prize winner, a guy with a girl, and a fabulous beast to look after as well. That night he hardly slept a wink.

Life was definitely on the up for Ben. He had helped to mentor Tim through to the Olympic Gold and his job at campus was going well. He was becoming a driving force in the crew.

The next day he phoned up Alex Davies at Collage and explained the situation. There was a moment's incredulity at the other end of the line, then "Awesome, man; congratulations! How do you fancy a party here at Collage?"

Ben had actually rung him for this purpose, so replied "Please Alex, that's what I had in mind, the crew and room for one more too –"

"Who could that be?" asked Alex.
"Oh, come off it – who could that be? Of course – he has four legs, wags his tail and is very hairy" Ben riddled.

"Leave it with me, Benbo, and I will get back to you on that one." Alex was non-committal there.

They rang off and Alex made out the point of a reservation, a table and a space for them all once again in his famous restaurant.

Ben felt to be on top of the world for a while. He knew not to let it go to his head, though – there was such a long way to go. So many improvements to be made, so many amendments and such a lot of editing to be done. The fun had only just begun.

Sure enough, on Wednesday at 11am there was a knock on the door. He had invited Suzanna, Tim, Alex, Shane, Claire, Charlie, Luke and his family round for the champagne celebration. His mum was a bit loopy herself and was keen to see the cheque in place in Ben's hands.

The two Camelot representatives came in to the living room with the camera, champagne and giant cheque. "Mr Williams – I believe this belongs to you," one of them said. "Many congratulations from Camelot".

Ben accepted the cheque graciously and then they went outside into the garden for photographs to be taken. Many pictures were taken of Ben, both individually and with the others too. A cork was popped and the champagne came gushing out of the bottle top soaking all those nearby.

Ben was asked what were his plans for the money. He said that he would hang onto most of it as a future investment. Some would be given to charity, either Dog's Trust, Macmillans, Blue Cross, Shelter, NSPCC, or British Heart Foundation, and the rest would be for spending, as of today, in restaurants, florists, and a holiday to Eastern Europe as well at some point not too far away. He also mentioned that he needed a new car too.

Everybody had a good laugh about the matter and chinked glasses. Within an hour Ben was recommended to call in the bank to cash the cheque, so he drove with Suzanna and Tim to HSBC and dealt with their business there.

Then all twelve people and the dog decided to make a move towards Collage. Alex had made an exception for this occasion. It was a celebration and should definitely be marked, so accordingly Collage had been pre-decorated with banners reading 'Congratulations, Ben' with balloons and streamers.

He may as well have won the jackpot for all the fuss that they were making over him, but for him it was a jackpot in itself. The evening rolled on and the two representatives disappeared first leaving the crew and Williams family to enjoy themselves. Pépé was under the table much of the time, chewing on some doggy drops or such like, out of the way. No one seemed to mind too much about the dog in the restaurant.

That was a time to behold for Ben Williams and co. One minute a break-in, the next a major prize. Good show, old chap. Pépé was on his best behaviour all night and seemed to know the score what was going on around him. He received some amicable tummy tickles and friendly pats from time to time.

The Williams star was shining now, all he had done was to match his numbers and he was now rich. He was glad to have got five and the bonus, which was a dramatic amount more than nought, one, or two. 'So much money for so little skill' he thought.

The afternoon wound down and the crew decided that a veritable result had been scored. Gradually they decided to call it a day and went on their way once again. Ben's parents wanted to know that he would pay them back their on-going two-grand debt that had been on the cards for three years now. He told them that he would now give them £250 every month for eight months, and they seemed happy with that arrangement, so he got out the cheque book there and then, knowing he was now in a good position financially. Though unable to move house, he would stick to it and who knows, maybe one day his life would change with another significant amount or more.

Anyway, that was that. An experience, and richer for it. Again, another sleepless night for Ben, tossing and turning wondering what would life be like with six matching numbers on the ticket. Oh well, he would have to make do with that he thought to himself.

And make do he did. He arranged for £85,000 to be deposited in a High Interest Deposit Bond with an interest rate of 8.5%. He opened two cash mini ISA, depositing £3,600 – the year's current maximum rate – into each of them, and he bought £25,000 worth of shares on the Alternative Investment Market...shares ranging in price from ½ pence to 3 pence per share. He figured that if these smaller companies thrived and their shares doubled in value to say 1pence, 2 pence, or God forbid 6 pence, then he would make at least a £50,000 killing within a 36 month period.

He decided to give almost 10% to charity. That would be well over £12,000, so he set up accounts with a dozen or so benevolent causes including education, health, accommodations, third world funds and music, art, and sporting donations too. Ben felt willing to contribute to those in greater need than himself. He would be a patron in this sense.

It was a bit of a gamble, but Ben figured that he could now afford to take this risk with his money. He had previously read magazines from Fleet Street's 'Red Hot Penny Share' quota and consulted an Independent Financial Advisor about such an investment. He also figured that if these shares thrived he may later apply to a Blue Chip company for a share portfolio of greater value.

Suzanna had advised him that he may as well go ahead with these dealings. The rest of the money ie over £65,000 went into his current account. Of that money, £12,000 was reserved for travelling at a later date; he hoped to go to Eastern Europe, maybe Latvia, Estonia, or Slovakia for a complete break. He didn't even speak Russian or any of the native tongues but was curious now that they were a part of the European Union. He also contemplated travelling to Australia, Singapore, Sweden or the USA.

He considered updating his vehicle. An inexpensive jalopy could now be improved upon. Room for two? Yes please, Ben. Maybe a few home improvements as well, a bit of a designer garden and some new furniture, furnishings, new room colour – maybe wallpaper in the living room, though he preferred a contemporary image by design. Mainly he hoped to create enough revenue so as to buy a city apartment and a continental villa to live in during the summer months. This would have to wait for the next instalment. The money in the Bond would eventually go towards a new property of some kind or other.

He treated some staff colleagues to a round of drinks one evening at the campus bar. There were those who were happy and those who were slightly envious, but those present were grateful for the drink. Ben had decided not to make too much of a big thing about his win.

Pépé was treated to a year's supply of biscuits, dog sausages, bones and assorted toys. Even a new basket cushion or three. They were chuffed now. Shane had no longer the same hatred towards Ben. Having spent their time together in London, and seeing both his sister's new rapport and Ben's success Shane had come round to accepting Ben into his conscious thoughts of being a friend, or at least, not a sworn mortal enemy as could have been the perception in earlier years.

Ben figured that his Pépé was as good a lucky mascot as could ever be found. Just as the Bradford team had their Bulls, Leeds their Rhinos, London their Wasps, Comic Relief its Pudsey bear, Ben had his Pépé dog – the loyalest Cocker Spaniel that could ever be found.

Suzanna was his, now. Claire was with Charlie; Alex and Melanie had been around for years now, with their daughter Fiona. 'Growing up fast, just too fast,' thought Alex and his wife. They had established an immaculate enterprise twice over between them and now the crew were pulling in new results over again.

Ben had decided to contact Tim once again to see how the new training regime was going on. Tim was more than happy for him and said that life had changed so much since London in the summer. He had been offered training schedules in foreign countries to experience climate changes, and changes in altitude where less oxygen appears in the air. So far, Tim had trained in Spain, Austria, France and Sweden on various triathlon courses, in lakes, in swimming pools, in the sea and, of course, on the hills as well to keep his legs good and strong.

Ben could no longer be his official mentor; there was no love lost between the two colleagues. The circumstances had changed so much over the last few years. It would come as no surprise that Tim had met his match in the competitive arena and was so absorbed with his training that life in Scarborough had really taken a back seat for the time being. He had international objectives and had had so for quite some time now.

Ben was so occupied with the work at Scarborough campus that this loss of position caused him no nostalgia. He had fought hard to gain it in the first place, but seeing the result, that had been the reward in itself for Ben. He needed no further confirmation, or acknowledgement of that role in particular. Life had brought forth the goods, so to speak.

Time pressed on. The crew, although separated in their own ways, were united in spirit. Events such as these brought them all together in person. They had come a long way since they first met. So much water had passed beneath the bridge, so much ground had been covered by these seven characters. Suddenly nothing seemed impossible.

Chapter 18
Collage

"Tell us a joke, Charlie", provoked Claire as they were all sat round the table in Collage wondering what to say.

"Alright, I will tell you a joke," said Charlie. "Here goes: a man walks into a bar and sees that the room is particularly crowded that evening. Se he walks towards the wall and places his hand against it. Then, he walks up the side of the wall, across the ceiling, and down the wall at the far side of the bar where he orders a pint of Tetley's Bitter. By this point, people are looking at him out of amazement and curiosity. The man proceeds to drink his pint then gives the barman a tip. He then returns to the wall, walks up it, across the ceiling, down the far-side wall and out the door to go home. A few mystified people looked at each other and said to the barman – 'that was a bit strange wasn't it'. The barman replied – 'yes, he normally orders a pint of Guinness!'".

Everyone chuckled at that joke. Claire was suitably impressed, then turned and asked everyone else: "OK, who else has got a good joke to tell us?"

Silence for a moment, then Suzanna coughed to gain composure and offered a number. "I know a joke," she said, "it goes a bit like this: set in Ireland at a Catholic convent school for girls, run by nuns. One year at the end of term all the final year leavers were gathered round and at the nuns' request were talking about what they would like to do upon leaving school. At first, one student came forwards and said 'sister, I would like to be an air hostess and see the world', to which the nun replied 'very well then. That sounds like an exciting occupation.' Then the next student came forwards and said 'sister, I would like to be a teacher in a college', and she replied 'most respectable indeed'. The third student came up and said 'sister, I would like very much to be a Director of a major organization'. She replied 'my, you are ambitious aren't you!' Then finally one student came forwards and said 'sister, you know – I've been thinking – I think I would like to be a prostitute'. The nun replied 'Oh thank God for that – for a moment I thought you were going to say Protestant'".

There was a pause as the punch line sank in then they got the joke. Suddenly the prospect of having a laugh kicked in, and other members began to recollect gags that they knew of. Ben decided to contribute next at the behest of Suzanna.

"Another man-in-a-bar joke", he said. "OK – a man walks into a bar one evening and orders a pint of his 'usual'. The barman complied with this request and then went out the back for a breath of fresh air. As the fellow proceeded to enjoy his beverage he heard a voice next to him saying 'Oi mister – you're a handsome devil aren't you; I like your jacket, your shirt and trousers. Bet you'd look better still underneath though - mmmmmm'. As he attempted to locate where the voice was coming from he could only see a bowl of peanuts on the bar table. Nobody else was present. So he felt perplexed for a moment and continued to enjoy his 'usual'. Then suddenly, another voice coming from the far end of the room: 'Oi dirtbag – get your ass out of here before I kick it out. Go back where you bloody well came from!' Again, he looked but saw noone, just a cigarette machine. Now he began to worry, so when the barman came back in he explained what he had heard, and the barman replied 'Oh, don't worry sir – the nuts are complementary, the cigarette machine is out of order'".

A contribution from Ben. Tim was in stitches at this point. Claire came up with two next: "Knock knock" – "who's there" – "Isabelle" – "Isabelle who?" – "Isabelle necessary on a bike". Then she apologised and offered another: "What is the definition of a clown giving a piggy back to a nun? – virgin on the ridiculous!"

"That's a good one C – I like it," commended Charlie.
"Yeah, that's real funny," said Suzanna.
"Anymore takers?" asked Tim. "I can hardly breathe for laughing", he said out loud. "Them's are good uns!"

Alex thought hard and suddenly remembered a bad school boy joke he had heard one time. "Do you remember the Englishman, Irishman, Scotchman jokes?" he asked generally.

"Oh no, not one of those" Melanie groaned.

"Yes, one of those" replied Alex. "Well, seeing as though we are onto jokes, here it is: there was an Englishman, an Irishman, and a Scotchman and they were being chased in a forest by bandits. Quickly they decided to each climb a tree to hide. The bandits were lost for a moment then they thought they had found them. So they went up to the first tree and shouted up 'is there anybody up there? Come down at once or we will shoot you down.' The Englishman made the noise of a bird calling. Then they said 'Oh, it is nothing – just a bird' and walked off to the next tree. Same again: 'is there anybody up there? Come down at once or we will shoot you down.' This time the Scotchman screeched like a monkey. 'Oh it is nothing, just a monkey', and they walked away to the next tree. This time they shouted out 'Come down at once if you are up there. You are surrounded.' At which point the Irishman said 'Mooooo'." Needless to say the end result.

"No offence to the Irish though", said Alex quickly.
"God, that was awful," scorned Shane, who hadn't told any jokes that evening.
"Well, you do better then – mate," demanded Alex.
"Nah, I prefer just to listen," Shane concluded.

They had had a decent round amongst themselves, and sat back feeling reasonably contented. They were in Collage again, the crew, all together and thinking about their journeys both past, and future. It seemed like an opportunity to compare notes once again and recollect what they had been through together, reminiscing.

Ben revelled in his status now and sparked up: "Just as the great maestro said, you have to elaborate to accumulate".

"That's a fine philosophy Benbo," said Suzanna. "I like it, to think that a snowball begins palm-sized and if rolled determinedly, ends man-sized".

"Yes, and that's not to mention hay-bailing. One field might produce one hundred bails, or more. If the farmer comes to harvest at the right time in the right way, that is", Charlie chipped in.

"You're such a scream man," laughed Alex.

"I wasn't trying to be funny," Charlie protested.

"You're a funny guy, Charlie Morris," Alex insisted.

They grinned mysteriously for a moment. Then Claire picked up on Ben's original point "You mean like writing songs for an album. One song does not an album make – it is cumulative. One requires at least a dozen tunes for the disc. At least an hour's music in all."

"Yes, Claire", replied Ben courteously, "I think you are picking up fast on this point. It would seem that you knew this long ago anyway, before you thought about it in the first place this evening."

"That's a bit long-winded," she gasped in exasperation.

"Well, that would be my game", Ben explained.

Again, another smile and a chuckle around the table, then all eyes were on Alex as he offered to bring out some bites to nibble at. There were olives, pitta bread and humous, cheeses, and some cold smoked ham to go at. Drinks were topped up once again, and they remained calm, happy, and appreciative that they could be together once again as before.

Alex commended everyone in turn: "It is not every day that Olympians, lottery winners, music stars, and future movers and shakers can all be together in the same place. For that reason I would like to propose a toast to us."

"To us", they all echoed, and took a swig.

"Yes, to us and the ends of time", joked Shane. That was his contribution to the evening. Suzanna smiled, suitably impressed with this.

"We should be alright for another while at least", hoped Charlie. "Time is as time does".

"An eternal dilemma, no beginning and no end, always was and always will be. Time is beyond mankind's control, although a manmade concept. If the universe came from nothing, what of the idea that 'nothing is something'", Ben philosophised.

"You mean like the inside of a tennis ball? Air pressure exists, although invisible to the naked eye. You can feel it, breathe it, but you will never get to see it – just the effects it causes on the surface," Shane piped up once again.

Ben turned to him and continued "You've got it man. The simplicity of it is disarming. Like electricity, you don't need to see it to believe it exists. The current says it all whether one understands, believes, or otherwise acknowledges it. The principles are the same for everyone – like gravity."
"Water flows downstream, ending in ponds, lakes, the sea, or the ocean. If you go with the flow you'll end up out in the open, but if you go against the current you'll have a rough ride. Like plaining across the grain of a piece of wood, rather than with the length of the grain", Claire mentioned. "Maybe it is sometimes necessary in order to get the end result that you require though", she added.

"New Balance, Nike, Reebok, Asics – they are more than just brands alone" said Tim. "We have to train in mind, body and spirit, to be the best we possibly can. The goddess of victory planned not commerce, but excellence on the field. We all see today so many by-products, so much high street retailing, so much fuel for the fire, so many drawn in. What we really require is the ability to formulate organic products and occurrences. Real events, this is what the world needs and thrives on."

The others took this point on board and remained sat round together. "Either way, as the great Bruce Hornsby said – the show goes on, that's just the way it is", Charlie included.

"Thanks Chaz", Claire said with gratitude.

"It's all good," said Alex quietly.

Ben had decided to produce some surprises with his available funds. He reached into his bag and one by one he handed out small gifts to each member as a milestone and to remember him by. A blue wristband for everyone with the words 'Ethics is alive' printed on.

Also, individual gifts too: Alex received a new watch, Melanie received a piece of artwork, Fiona a doll, Claire and Charlie were given a couple of CD's – one jazz singing, the other folk music – Luke was there too and handed a toy action hero; Suzanna was given a hug and a box of chocolates, Shane given Al Gore's book 'An inconvenient truth', and Tim was given his own signed photograph as he crossed the finish line at the London Games of 2012 – it was at least framed and Ben had written a presentation card to go along with it.

Everybody was surprised and grateful for this move all of a sudden. It would mean a lot to them that Ben had made a special effort for each of them. As for his dog, Pépé, he would be at home with an extra bone to chew on. Ben would enjoy the company when he returned later. Alex never did concur to allowing the dog inside. This would have caused something of a customer discrepancy amongst the other guests there in Collage.

Suddenly Alex said to them "Guys, I have to nip across to the café to check up on something, I will be back soon – don't go without me." He then proceeded to leave them for less than an hour and walk to The Flaming Squirrels to check up on the accounts details. He was in credit as far as he could make out, so felt happy with that fact and then returned to Collage to join them once again.

There was a sense of expectation when he returned as if he were going to announce something fantastic. As it was he just had a quiet word with Melanie and told her what he had just confirmed. She already knew so told him that as well. They sat, glad to be above board in restaurant and café. Feeling privileged to be able to host such a gathering Alex shook Ben's hand and thanked him once again for the watch. He did not take such generosity lightly.

It meant a lot to him that he had such a friend who would share his good fortune with others. Ben was fortunate. Prosperity had shone upon him abundantly, and he was now able to use this to his advantage by purchasing some tokens of appreciation for his friends. His fortune was extended unto others as much as to gratify his own requirements. He had Suzanna to keep a check on things as well. She would direct him if needs be, like a rudder on a boat. A degree of difference now could make the entire journey bumpy or smooth.

He had hoped for a life of success and happiness so went out of the way to keep his friends. They meant a lot to him. He had almost got used to being a single, lonely bachelor until the point where he had met Suzanna and Pépé. He now had friends and they were good for him, causing more joy than consternation. At least they were a reliable bunch.

In the background there was some cool jazz playing on the restaurant sound system. There was a female vocalist with band – piano, drums, bass, saxophone and guitar for various tracks. It was a combination of mellow music and frenetic, uptempo entertainment. Claire revelled in the music played and made note to inquire about the artist and track titles. Alex ended up lending her the disc to take home.

"Thanks man – I'll enjoy this beauty like an orchid coming in to bloom on a summer's day", she told Alex at that point.

"So long as that's a promise", he answered.

Charlie smiled briefly then asked Claire who the CD was of. "Oh, it's Clare Teale on vocals", she told him. "She is the UK's most dynamic performer today", she went on. "Jazz artiste suprema to be honest", she commended the musician. "Must do credit to the likes of Tom Cawley as well. Not to mention Julie Edwards, Kevin Dearden, Jamil Sheriff, Claire Martin, Courtney Pine, Alcyona Mick, or Guy Barker – to name but a few", she elaborated a little.

In truth there were so many bands around that to name any of them would mean discrediting so many others. There had been a recent festival in Scarborough with music and punters of all isms and schisms attending. All genders, ages, races and other agendas to keep. Claire and Charlie had attended, she had hoped for a gig, but the lineup went to other artists on the day. She was happy to even be present to listen with him.

Nobody would ever have denied her the opportunity for Seachimp to perform but the festival organisers decreed that 'no band shall perform two years running'. Seachimp had already performed previously so were thus ruled out of this year's showing. A logical sequence of events all in all. Sherlock Holmes would be proud of the logic: 'elementary dear Watson'.

Maybe the whole procedure had been merely elementary, not a complication in sight, just a string of occurrences and characterful happenings. But what did they care? For Claire, Charlie, Shane, Suzanna, Ben, Tim and Alex they were glad of one another, even though their paths had taken on dramatically different directions over the years. They were connected somehow, and not just by Orange, 3, O2, Vodafone, or T-Mobile, but by spirit, emotion and events leading up to the present moment. In time for another, they thought.

Whether that would be good or bad, happy or sad, great or small, long, short, or tall – that remained to be seen. All they knew for now was that here and now they were together in Collage celebrating their unity by diversity. That said a lot without even saying anything at all.

Something that Tim could specialise in – he often said things by his actions alone and left the talking to the rest of the world. His fitness spoke volumes and nobody here wanted to jeopardise this reality for him. Actuality for Tim remained a long shot for Shane. His accomplishments had mounted up over a period of time and now had amounted to something significant. An Olympic medal and a whole host of local victories on various courses. He was deservedly pleased now, although not looking back at all. Tim was holding onto his vision for a faster, fitter future.

Alex was holding onto his own vision as well, for the profitable, venturing days to continue. He intended to remain above water as far as he could possibly help it. At this moment in time, it all looked more than likely. He was getting the custom and people liked his place. Melanie and Fiona had helped grow it all up as well; they were an integral factor to these establishments.

Charlie too had his venture to care for. Owner and father of one, he was careful to respect others now as he had a lot to lose if he went over the line once again. Claire helped him see to it that he remained on top of the game. She was almost businesslike with the song productions, churning out numbers on a regular basis.

Ben desired Suzanna more than ever now. They had really been through the mill together since they first met, and now their relationship was blooming. The sun had risen above the waterline and the orange orb was glowing effusively in the sky for all to see. The others could get warm just thinking about this. It was something of an establishment in itself.

Charlie Morris wanted the best for himself and his own. What this might mean was that he had to make sacrifices along the way. Whether to spend quality time with Claire and Luke, or whether to arrange a day trip some place else, he had to account for a lot of factors en route.

Singing his praises often, Claire felt alive to be in his company. They had saved each other from eternal obscurity, and entered a new world of meaning. Neither had known what to expect since then but the outcome so far was favourable. Charlie liked to think that he was top dog here. Claire never took that away from him. She loved him.

"I've still been thinking about Megan and Darren since they lost Henry. Maybe I should go and make a personal visit and see if I can bring some better news for them?" said Claire.

"Oh, I don't know C; Sometimes you just have to leave a tender moment alone", replied Charlie.

"I always knew her so well though. It would be out of duty more than anything", she went on.

"I guess you should do whatever you feel best for you and them. There is no bringing back Henry now whatever you say or do", said Charlie harshly.

"That's precisely what I mean. I could be the 'old friend' coming back again. Anyway, I'm sure Megan wouldn't want an unwelcome intrusion once again", Claire concluded.

With that they sat back in their seats thoughtfully for a while.

Suddenly it was the time again to go their different ways at the end of the evening. But there was still time before they left. Tim had a call from Vinny by chance, telling him that a new meet had been called in Manchester next season on the bike. Tim was interested to hear the news and told him he was with some friends back home. Their call didn't last long though. Back to the crew, there were due regards and homage to be paid to one another. Nobody wanted to say goodbye this time, as it was a one night only affair. The end of the night was in sight. To keep them together, Ben offered to show a film at his place. A Ben Stiller/Jack Black comedy – he had the complete collection at home. At first there was some interest expressed, but on the whole it was going to be a Collage send-off.

So there they were at this point after their travels so far. "What do you say we have a game of twister?" stated Suzanna......"you know, boys and girls getting tied in knots together on the floor kind-a-thing".

The all laughed with mirth at that. Alex informed them that they were out of fresh twisters at the moment so would have to come up with something else instead. Ben came up with another suggestion: "Pépé requires dog duty tonight – any volunteers?"

"That'll be your realm Benbo – best leave that to you sir" said Alex. Then Suzanna suddenly chirped up "I'll walk with you love" she offered nobly.

"Thanks sweetheart, I would appreciate that," Ben returned.

And with that it was time. Ben and Suzanna got up to get their jackets on and went round each crew member shaking hands and embracing, wishing everyone their warmest wishes before taking off into the night. They then vacated the premises and left for reasons of responsibility.

Claire went outside to smoke a cigarette. Meanwhile, Charlie, Alex, Shane and Tim stayed in talking amongst themselves in a low key fashion. They were glad of the occasion and accepted that it may be some time before they were to meet again. Shane made reference to the other guys about being a sole agent, a warrior of the night, a lone ranger. Alex told him to keep at it, somebody had to. It wasn't the end of the world after all.

Tim got up next and said that he was back to training early the next morning so may as well leave now. He thanked Alex for the hospitality and gave the lads a high five each with a comment too. He then put on his sports jacket and went to leave Collage. As he left, Alex shouted out "may the force be with you my friend – let it be magnificent."

Tim saluted and then went out into the night to go home. He passed Claire outside and gave her a quick hug and then went.

She came back inside and sat with Charlie. "You know what dude – I will miss Tim. He has been such an inspiration to us all. Every move, every word, every look; a source of motivation, wisdom and insight. He got lucky to know Ben when he did. I reckon that really improved his performance overall you know."

"Yeah, he's one movin', groovin' dude alright" replied Charlie. They sat in thought briefly then decided to follow suite and went to get their jackets. Alex called them over to him before the big send off.

Shane said "Well, it's that time I guess". He also stood up to leave on his own. He had enjoyed the evening, quiet as he was. Maybe there would be somebody, somewhere for Shane. Alex commended him for attending and then proceeded to shake his hand and said to call in again soon.

So this was the end for the crew. A pleasant time with all and sundry present. Melanie had come back to help Alex clear up the place. It needed very little doing on this occasion. Not too many other people had come in tonight, so it was a half hour job to shut up shop.

So that was that. The crew had come together, they had performed, been through storm, wind and weather and now were moving on once again. In a reflective moment, Alex grabbed a poetry book and flipped it open at a random page. The poem was by Stevie Smith and he read it out to Melanie, "In my dreams – In my dreams I am always saying goodbye and riding away, whither and why I know not nor do I care. And the parting is sweet and the parting over is sweeter, and sweetest of all is the night and the rushing air."

"In my dreams they are always waving their hands and saying goodbye, and they give me the stirrup cup and I smile as I drink, I am glad the journey is set, I am glad I am going, I am glad, I am glad, that my friends don't know what I think."

It seemed to be appropriate to the moment as the evening had concluded. Melanie said it was great and took a turn. She located an Elizabeth Jennings verse called 'Friendship'. She told Alex she had chosen it for him. "Such love I cannot analyse; it does not rest in lips or eyes, neither in kisses nor caress. Partly, I know, it's gentleness and understanding in one word or in brief letters. It's preserved by trust and by respect and awe. These are the words I'm feeling for. Two people, yes, two lasting friends. The giving comes, the taking ends. There is no measure for such things. For this all nature slows and sings."

A beautiful verse and Alex simply went to her and wrapped her in his arms. They stood there as the lights were low. Next they would see a new chapter, a new dawn and a new day. Either way they were glad for what they had been through.

One thing was for sure – they would have to stick at it, keep ploughing the furrow and reshaping their plans. Plan 103f had been for them. The original concepts had come, life had thrown down the gauntlet for them, they bit the bullet, and now they were back to themselves once again. This was just the beginning.

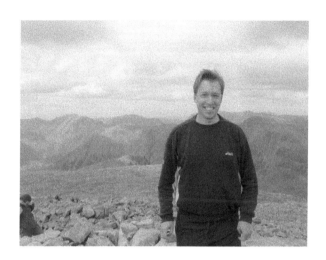